Psychopathology and Violent Crime

EDITED BY
Andrew E. Skodol, M.D.

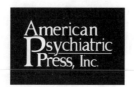

WASHINGTON, DC
LONDON, ENGLAND

Copyright © 1998 American Psychiatric Press, Inc.
First Edition 01   00   99   98   4   3   2   1
ALL RIGHTS RESERVED
Manufactured in the United States of America on acid-free paper

American Psychiatric Press, Inc.
1400 K Street, N.W.
Washington, DC   20005
www.appi.org

Library of Congress Cataloging-in-Publication Data

Psychopathology and violent crime / edited by Andrew E. Skodol.
    p.   cm.
    Includes bibliographical references and index.
    ISBN 0-88048-834-4 (alk. paper)
    1. Criminals—Mental health.   2. Violence—Psychological aspects.
  3. Psychology, Pathological.   I. Skodol, Andrew E.
  RC451.4.P68P68 1998
  616.89'0086'927—dc21   97-51790
                                                                      CIP

British Library Cataloguing in Publication Data

A CIP record is available from the British Library.

Contents

Contributors

Paul S. Appelbaum, M.D. A. F. Zeleznik Distinguished Professor and Chair, Department of Psychiatry, and Director, Law and Psychiatry Program, University of Massachusetts Medical School, Worcester, Massachusetts

James C. Beck, M.D., Ph.D. Associate Chair, Department of Psychiatry, Cambridge Hospital; and Associate Professor, Consolidated Department of Psychiatry, Harvard Medical School, Boston, Massachusetts

Emil F. Coccaro, M.D. Professor of Psychiatry, Clinical Neuroscience Research Unit, Department of Psychiatry, MCP Hahnemann School of Medicine, Allegheny University of the Health Sciences, Philadelphia, Pennsylvania

Jeremy W. Coid, M.D., F.R.C.Psych. Professor of Forensic Psychiatry, Academic Section of Forensic Psychiatry, St. Bartholomew's and the Royal London School of Medicine and Dentistry, London, United Kingdom

Brian McNamee, M.D., J.D. Formerly Clinical Instructor, Case Western Reserve School of Medicine, Cleveland, Ohio

John M. Oldham, M.D. Director, New York State Psychiatric Institute; and Professor and Vice Chairman, Department of Psychiatry, Columbia University College of Physicians and Surgeons, New York, New York

Michelle B. Riba, M.D. Clinical Associate Professor of Psychiatry and Associate Chair for Education and Academic Affairs, Department of Psychiatry, University of Michigan Health System, Ann Arbor, Michigan

Andrew E. Skodol, M.D. Professor of Clinical Psychiatry, Columbia University College of Physicians and Surgeons; and Director, Department of Personality Studies, New York State Psychiatric Institute, New York, New York

Michael H. Stone, M.D. Professor of Clinical Psychiatry, Columbia University College of Physicians and Surgeons, New York, New York; and Staff Psychiatrist, MidHudson Psychiatric Center, New Hampton, New York

Heidi Wencel, M.A. Fellow in Neuropsychology, Department of Psychiatry, Cambridge Hospital; and Clinical Fellow, Harvard Medical School, Boston, Massachusetts

Introduction to the Review of Psychiatry Series

John M. Oldham, M.D., and Michelle B. Riba, M.D.,
Series Editors

Beginning with 1998, the annual Review of Psychiatry adopts a new format. What were individual sections bound together in a large volume will be published only as independent monographs. Each monograph provides an update on a particular topic. Readers may then selectively purchase those monographs of particular interest to them. Last year, Volume 16 was available in the large volume and individual monographs, and the individually published sections were immensely successful. We think this new format adds flexibility and convenience to the always popular series.

Our goal is to maintain the overall mission of this series—that is, to provide useful and current clinical information, linked to new research evidence. For 1998 we have selected topics that overlap and relate to each other: 1) Psychopathology and Violent Crime, 2) New Treatments for Chemical Addictions, 3) Psychological Trauma, 4) Biology of Personality Disorders, 5) Child Psychopharmacology, and 6) Interpersonal Psychotherapy. All of the editors and chapter authors are experts in their fields. The monographs capture the current state of knowledge and practice while providing guideposts to future lines of investigation.

We are indebted to Helen ("Sam") McGowan for her dedication and skill and to Linda Gacioch for all of her help. We are indebted to the American Psychiatric Press, Inc., under the leadership of Carol C. Nadelson, M.D., who has supported this important and valued review series. We thank Claire Reinburg, Pamela Harley, Ron McMillen, and the APPI staff for all their generous assistance.

Foreword

Andrew E. Skodol, M.D.

A recent article in the *New York Times* reported that rates of serious crime across the nation including murder, rape, robbery, aggravated assault, burglary, and larceny have decreased by approximately 10% over the past 5 years (Butterfield 1997). Lest Americans become complacent about crime, however, the article went on to state that, over the same interval, the number of prison inmates in the United States has grown by almost 45%.

One simple explanation, therefore, for the observed reduction in crime is that, with more persons convicted of crime given prison sentences and more kept in prison longer, fewer potential criminals are free in the community, able to commit crimes. This might appear to be a tidy solution to the problem of serious crime in this country, except when the costs of imprisonment are considered. In the state of California, which has seen its prison population grow eightfold in the last two decades, it costs almost six times as much per year to house a prisoner as it does to educate a child in the State University system. California, which has both the highest number of prison inmates in the country and a state law that caps government revenue, now spends more to incarcerate people than it does to educate its college-age children. In addition to the direct costs of prisons for perpetrators of serious crime, indirect social costs result from the disruption of family structure and the creation of criminal subcultures that result from prolonged imprisonment.

The costs of violent crime to victims, in terms of loss, pain, suffering, and death are also great. Firearm injuries alone kill 40,000 persons and harm another 240,000 in the United States each year (American Medical Association 1995). Firearm injuries rival motor vehicle accidents as the leading cause of unnatural death in the United States, are the eighth leading cause of death overall, and are the fourth leading cause of death for the population under 65 (Annest et al. 1995). The mean hospital cost for treating a firearm-related injury has been estimated at more than $52,000; the median cost at more than $28,000 (Kizer et al. 1995). The estimated cost for providing for medical care for such injuries in the United States in 1995 was $4 billion and the total estimated direct and indirect costs of firearm injuries were $14 billion.

Finally, the costs of violent crime to potential victims, in terms of fear, anxiety, paranoia, and isolation, cannot be underestimated. A recent study reported that 40% of 6th, 8th, and 10th graders in an urban setting had been exposed to a shooting or a stabbing in the past year (Schwab-Stone et al. 1995). Seventy-four percent reported feeling unsafe in one or more common environments: home, neighborhood, school, or on the way to school. Violence exposure was related to greater willingness to use physical aggression, diminished perceptions of risk of activities, lowered personal expectations for the future, dysphoric mood, antisocial activity, alcohol use, and decreased school achievement. Clearly, the economic and social costs of violent crime threaten to overwhelm our capacity to absorb them.

The relationship between mental disorder and serious violent crime is both controversial and complex. Despite media portrayals and popular opinion to the contrary, studies of patients with mental disorders and of prison inmates conducted before the 1990s failed to show any increased risk of violent crime among persons with mental disorders (Monahan and Steadman 1984). Now, however, as the end of the decade approaches, a sea change seems to have occurred. As data have accumulated from recent epidemiologic samples of community residents, as well as from more rigorous studies of criminal populations, a consensus is emerging that violent crime and mental disorder are strongly linked.

The reasons for this dramatic shift in professional opinion and its implications for society are as yet unclear. Methodologically superior studies; more comprehensive concepts of mental disorder; increases in the incidence of high-risk mental disorders, such as substance use disorders; or real increases in the rate at which persons with mental disorder commit crimes may each contribute to the strengthened associations found. Whether these findings should influence judicial deliberations on culpability, sentencing considerations, treatment approaches, or preventative efforts remains to be seen.

In this book, chapters review new data on the relationship of violent crime to Axis I psychopathology, on violent crime and personality disorders, on genetic and neurobiological studies of aggression, and on the implications of these findings for the legal system. Important questions addressed include the magnitude of the association between psychopathology and violent crime; the extent of violent crime accounted for by persons with mental disorders, including substance use disorders; the motivations for crime in the mentally ill; biological, psychological, and social factors influencing violence in those with mental disorders; the role of psychiatric treatment in managing violent offenders; and the significance of the association of violent crime and psychopathology for the criminal justice and penal systems and for the prevention of violent crime.

In the opening chapter of the book, James Beck and Heidi Wencel review the recent explosion of studies on the relationship of Axis I mental disorders and violence since 1990. Their chapter is organized by method of sample selection, presenting epidemiologic studies, studies of persons charged with or convicted of violent crimes, and studies of persons with mental disorders who commit violent crimes. They discuss the role of delusions in the genesis of violent behavior among psychotic persons. And finally, they discuss the roles of and interactions between brain dysfunction and social deficits, including low socioeconomic status (SES), family dysfunction, and inadequate parenting, on the genesis of violent behavior.

An interest in Axis II psychopathology in violent offenders is relatively new. It has long been accepted that antisocial personality disorder (ASPD), almost by definition, could be associated with violent crime. But, since reliable measurement of other Axis II disorders was not possible before their definition by diagnostic criteria in DSM-III (American Psychiatric Association 1980) and the subsequent development of semistructured interviews for their assessment, they were often overlooked in relationship to violence. In the second chapter, Michael Stone vividly and convincingly argues for the importance not only of ASPD but also of other personality psychopathology, including psychopathy, narcissism, sadism, and borderline psychopathology, in understanding some of society's most horrific murderers. Stone weaves together research data, his own clinical experience as a forensic psychiatrist, and a unique distillation of personality profiles from the biographies of almost 300 murderers to make the case for the importance of personality in the motivation to kill and in considering the prognosis of those who have murdered.

Jeremy Coid continues with the theme of Axis II psychopathology and violent crime, based on his research in the prisons and maximum security hospitals in the United Kingdom. The U.K. judicial approach to violent crime differs from that in the United States, in that violent offenders are more likely to receive psychiatric examinations. Mental health laws in the United Kingdom discourage the incarceration of psychotic persons in ordinary prisons, but allow for the preventative detainment of persons believed to be dangerous to society in special secure hospitals. Coid has previously demonstrated that ASPD is highly prevalent among men in U.K. prisons and secure hospitals and that borderline personality disorder (BPD) is highly prevalent among women. In this chapter, he presents a typology of motivation for violent crime and a study linking Axis I and Axis II disorders to the motivations for violent crime.

In the fourth chapter of the book, Emil Coccaro and Brian McNamee link together psychopathology and violent, aggressive behavior at the neurobiological level. First, they review evidence from twin and adoption studies for a genetic component to criminal behavior. Then, they present the rapidly expanding data on the roles of neurotransmitter mediators, such as serotonin, norepinephrine, and dopamine and of metabolic and hormonal mediators, such as glucose, testosterone, and cholesterol, in crime and aggression. Finally, they conclude with a case study of a man accused of murder for whom the results of biological studies were presented at trial as part of a criminal defense plea of not guilty by reason of insanity. This interesting case—and its outcome—sets the stage for the final chapter of the book.

The law has a long history of attempting to deal with the relationship of crime and mental disorder. Paul Appelbaum traces this history, beginning with Aristotle's argument that confusion about the reality of a situation might provide a moral excuse for persons who acted unlawfully in response to their beliefs. Appelbaum considers the implications for the law if violent crime were shown to be clearly linked to mental disorder and, further, if someday biological factors at the individual level could be shown to be a cause of violent behavior. Would such individuals be exculpated from responsibility for their acts, treated instead of punished, confined only for as long as they required secure circumstances for treatment? Should any of these revisions in the criminal justice or penal systems occur? Appelbaum presents the pros and cons of such changes and argues that both history and common sense should induce skepticism in the reader.

This book, though presenting cutting-edge research and clinical wisdom on violence and psychopathology, will probably raise as many questions as it answers. Nonetheless, these chapters demonstrate that psychiatry continues to make strides in combating one of our nation's most serious public health problems (Koop and Lundberg 1992).

References

American Medical Association: Medical news and perspectives. JAMA 273:1739–1740, 1995

American Psychiatric Association: Diagnostic and Statistical Manual of Mental Disorders, 3rd Edition. Washington, DC, American Psychiatric Association, 1980

Annest JL, Mercy JA, Gibson DR, et al: National estimates of nonfatal firearm-related injuries: beyond the tip of the iceberg. JAMA 273:1749–1754, 1995

Butterfield F: Punitive damages: crime keeps on falling, but prisons keep on filling. New York Times, September 28, 1997, Section 4, pp 1, 4

Kizer KW, Vassar MJ, Harry RL, et al: Hospitalization charges, costs, and income for firearm-related injuries at a university trauma center. JAMA 273:1768–1773, 1995

Koop CE, Lundberg GD: Violence in America: a public health emergency. JAMA 267:3075–3076, 1992

Monahan J, Steadman HJ: Crime and Mental Disorder. Washington, DC, National Institute of Justice, Research in Brief, September, 1984

Schwab-Stone ME, Ayers TS, Kasprow W, et al: No safe haven: a study of violence exposure in an urban community. J Am Acad Child Adolesc Psychiatry 34:1343–1352, 1995

Chapter 1

Violent Crime and Axis I Psychopathology

James C. Beck, M.D., Ph.D., and Heidi Wencel, M.A.

In this chapter, we review an extraordinary recent outpouring of research on the relationship between violent crime and Axis I psychopathology. In so doing, we document a significant development in the intellectual history of psychiatry. In a brief time, no more than 5 to 7 years, two major changes in thinking have occurred. First, the revealed wisdom of a generation that held that crime and mental disorder were unrelated has been rejected. Second, and even more unusual, this belief has been replaced by its opposite. The now substantial evidence that violent crime and Axis I psychopathology are meaningfully related to each other has been accepted.

Since antiquity a relationship between mental disorder and violence has been observed. In 1 Samuel, the author wrote, "an evil spirit from God rushed upon Saul, and he raved within his house . . . and Saul had his spear in his hand. And Saul cast the spear, for he thought, "I will pin David to the wall" (1 Samuel 18:10–11). In Euripides' retelling of the myth of Hercules, Hercules became mad and killed his own and his brother's children (Euripides 1959).

Contemporary Americans have long associated mental illness and violence—an association encouraged by television programs that have often portrayed mentally ill characters as more violent than others (Signorelli 1989). Court opinions also reflected this belief. A California court opined in the 1960s, "On the assembly line or in the railroad shop, an adjacent known psychotic employee is no less dangerous than an adjacent known unsafe machine" (*Najera v. Southern Pacific Co.* 1961). Even the

Supreme Court equated mental illness and dangerousness. The Court held that a man found not guilty by reason of insanity was sufficiently dangerous to justify continued involuntary hospitalization. The man was mentally ill, but the only evidence of his dangerousness was that he had stolen a leather jacket (*Jones v. United States* 1983).

Prior to 1990, studies of the relationship between violent crime and mental disorder were methodologically inadequate to establish whether a relationship existed. There were studies of patient violence, patient arrest rates for violent crime, and persons detained in jails. Each of these types of studies is subject to biases that do not permit generalization to the population at large. Based on what little empirical work existed, however, two of the best researchers on violence and mental disorder in the country concluded, "The scant research into mental disorder among persons who have been arrested ('true criminals') suggests that their rates of disorder are no higher than those of the general American population of comparable social class" (Monahan and Steadman 1984). Their view accurately reflected psychiatric opinion until 1990.

This chapter reviews studies on the relationship of violence to Axis I mental disorders since 1990. It is organized by method of sample selection: 1) epidemiologic samples designed to represent an entire community or society; 2) samples of persons charged with or convicted of violent crimes; and 3) samples of persons with mental disorders. Every study that evaluated alcohol and substance use disorders has found a substantial relationship between substance use disorders and violent crime. This review addresses the more controversial relationship of other Axis I disorders and violent crime and will not repetitively report the consistent results for alcohol and substance use disorders, except as disorders comorbid with other Axis I psychopathology. The review concludes with mention of recent research on biological and social risk factors for violent behavior in the mentally ill. Other biological research, including genetic and neurotransmitter studies, is reviewed in Chapter 4, by Coccaro and McNamee.

Epidemiologic Studies

In 1990 Swanson et al. published the first epidemiologic data that linked mental disorder and violence. In the Epidemiologic Catchment Area (ECA) study, interviews with more than 10,000 people, scientifically sampled in three metropolitan areas, provided data on mental disorder and on self-reported violence in the past year. Between 10% and 12% of persons with affective or schizophrenic disorders reported having been violent as compared with 2% of persons with no mental disorders. Twenty-five percent of those with alcohol abuse and 35% of those with substance abuse also reported violent behavior.

Link, Cullen, and Andrews (1992) provided the second set of data that convincingly established a relationship between mental disorder and violence. They interviewed a sample of residents of one New York City neighborhood and a sample of neighborhood residents who were patients at the local mental health center. They obtained mental health histories and arrest records for their study participants, as well as demographic data and census data describing the neighborhood. Current and former patients had been arrested significantly more often for violent crimes than had other neighborhood residents, and they also reported using weapons more often during the past 5 years. These results held true, independent of relevant demographic characteristics of participants and neighborhood data. Last, going beyond patient status to specific psychopathology, the authors showed that individuals who self-reported violence also reported active delusional beliefs. This association was independent of whether the person was or was not a patient.

In a later study, Link and Steuve (1994) focused the significance of delusions even more sharply. They found that delusions of threat, as occur for example in paranoid schizophrenia or delusional disorder, or delusions of control, as occur in schizophrenia, such as thought insertion or the belief that someone is controlling one's thoughts, were associated with violence, but that other delusions were not.

Stating a theme to be kept in mind throughout this chapter,

Link et al. (1992) cautioned that the contribution of mental disorder to the total amount of community violence is trivial. They noted, for example, that census tract homicide rates alone predicted 60% of the variance in rates of violence between neighborhoods. Age, gender, and education were also more strongly associated with violence than was mental disorder. Swanson (1994) made a similar point, estimating that roughly 3% of violence in the community was perpetrated by persons with mental illness. Although mentally ill people are more violent than others, there are relatively few of them. As a practical matter, alcohol abuse makes a far larger contribution to American violence than all other mental disorders combined.

Danish record keeping is among the most complete in the world. Hodgins et al. (1996) made use of these records to study a cohort of 324,000 consecutive newborns from birth until the age of 43. Eleven thousand women and 10,000 men with a history of psychiatric hospitalization were compared with all others. Diagnoses were given hierarchically, so that each subject had just one. The hierarchy was 1) major mental disorder (MMD), 2) mental retardation, 3) organic mental disorder, 4) antisocial personality disorder (ASPD), 5) drug addiction, 6) alcoholism, and 7) other disorder. Thus, for example, anyone diagnosed with alcoholism had no diagnosis higher on the list.

Both men and women in all diagnostic groups except those with organic mental disorders were at higher risk of having been convicted of a violent crime than were persons with no mental disorder. The increased risk of violent crime was consistently higher for women than for men across all diagnostic groups. That is, mental disorder seemed to relate more strongly to violent crime in women than in men. The authors noted that the extent to which these findings generalized to other countries would depend on similarities in society, criminal justice, and health care institutions. One question this study could not address because of the method of assigning diagnosis was the extent to which substance abuse or antisocial personality in association with an MMD increased the risk of violent crime.

Widom and Maxfield (1996) compared 908 abused children with a set of 667 matched control subjects. Abused children had the highest rate of arrest as adults for violent crime, 18.2%, compared with 13.9% of control subjects (OR [odds ratio] = 1.35), a modest but significant difference. A logistic regression analysis showed that the following variables independently predicted arrest for violent crime: male gender (OR = 6.4), African American ethnic status (OR = 4.1), physical abuse (OR = 1.9), and neglect (OR = 1.55).

Studies of Violent Criminals

Murderers

Tiihonen (1993) reported on a study of all persons in Finland who were arrested for homicide from June 1990 to May 1991. Finnish police solved more than 94% of all homicides during this time, so this is a remarkably complete sample. One hundred and seven (98 men, 9 women) of 140 arrestees were referred for forensic psychiatric evaluation. The 33 nonreferred persons were assumed to be without psychiatric disorder, which may slightly bias the results toward an underestimate of the relationship of homicide and mental disorder. Base rates of mental disorder in the population were drawn from U.S. data (ECA), which are considered comparable to Finnish base rates. Among the men who committed homicide, schizophrenia was 6.5 times more prevalent than in the general population; among the few women it was 15 times more prevalent. Affective disorder was 1.8 times more prevalent in men, but no different for women. The authors noted a strong association of alcoholism and antisocial personality with homicide and, further, that these were type II early-onset alcoholic children of alcoholic fathers.

In a later study, the same group (Eronen et al. 1996a) reported on a sample of Finnish homicide offenders ($n = 693$) evaluated by a forensic team over 8 years. This sample represented approximately 77% of all Finnish homicide offenders. Adjusting for age, there were far more offenders with schizophrenia ($n = 63$) than would occur by chance (OR = 8.0). Offenders with alcoholism ($n = 384$) were also overrepresented (OR = 10.7), as were offenders with ASPD ($n = 114$) (OR $= 11.7$). There was a smaller effect for major depression (OR $= 1.6$). Offenders with dysthymia or anxiety disorders were represented at chance levels. The authors did not report data for patients with comorbid Axis I and II disorders, for example schizophrenia and ASPD. However, in another paper (Eronen et al. 1996b), the authors evaluated 1,423 homicide offenders and reported data for schizophrenia with and without alcoholism. Men with schizophrenia and alcoholism ($n = 38$) had ORs of greater than 17.0 for homicide compared with the general population; for men with schizophrenia alone ($n = 48$) the OR was greater than 7.0. For the very few women with schizophrenia (3 with alcoholism and 5 without) who murdered, the differences were even more extreme.

Another paper from the same group reported on the risk of homicide in 281 released forensic psychiatric patients (Tiihonen et al. 1996). The likelihood that these discharged patients with schizophrenia would commit a homicide was more than 50 times greater than the likelihood for the general population. Eronen et al. (1996c) identified 36 people who had killed again after being released from prison. Twenty-four were alcoholic and 23 of these had personality disorders. Four had schizophrenia (OR > 25.0 for committing a homicide compared with the general population).

Malmquist (1995) has reviewed literature and individual cases that also illustrated a relationship between depression with psychotic symptoms and violence or homicide.

Other Violent Defendants or Offenders

Steury and Choinski (1995) studied 114 men and their victims. The men had been charged with violent crimes in Milwaukee County between 1981 and 1985. The authors tested the commonly held belief that mentally deranged people attack strangers.

The crimes were homicide (38%), endangerment (32%), and battery (28%). Patient-defendants ($n = 32$) were defined as those who had a mental health contact within 2 years of arrest. Fifty percent of the patient-defendants were diagnosed with schizophrenia. The 32 patient-defendants were compared with the 82 men in the sample of 114 who had no such contact, and with all felony defendants in Milwaukee over the same time period. Patient-defendants were more likely to commit deadly and dangerous crimes than were other defendants. They were less likely to attack strangers (16%) than were control subjects (26%). Patient-defendant crimes were characterized as more often occurring in family arguments at home, unplanned or without apparent motive, not involving drugs or alcohol, and with intent to harm but not to kill. Other defendant crimes were characterized as occurring after prior trouble with the victim, were often motivated by a sign of disrespect or occurred during a robbery, and were the result of intent to kill. Patient-defendant weapons of choice were knives; other defendants used guns. Patient-defendants with a diagnosis of psychosis were especially likely to have used a knife during a trivial argument and without history of prior trouble—a so-called senseless crime. This study is unique in providing data on the relationship between defendant and victim and on the specifics of the criminal act. The results are in direct opposition to popular belief—the mentally ill preferentially killed family at home, not strangers elsewhere.

Martell et al. (1995) studied 184 criminal defendants diagnosed with mental disorder after forensic psychiatric evaluation in New York City. The authors found that 43% of defendants with mental disorders were homeless, compared with an estimated 2% of the population of New York City. Homeless defendants were 40 times more likely to have been charged with a violent crime than were domiciled defendants. The OR for murder equaled 25.0; for attempted murder, 60.0. Victims of homeless persons' crimes were strangers in 93% of cases, compared with 76% of domiciled persons' victims. This study documented a high rate of violent crime among homeless mentally ill defendants, in contrast to mentally ill defendants who had somewhere to live. The victims were far more often strangers than in the Milwaukee sample already discussed.

Repo et al. (1997) studied 282 arsonists who had received a forensic psychiatric evaluation, and compared first-time offenders with offenders who had a prior history of violent crime. These 282 represented only 10% of Finnish arsonists, so the sample was not representative. Twenty-seven percent of the first offenders were diagnosed with schizophrenia or delusional disorder, 12% with major mood disorder, 46% with alcohol dependence, 27% with minor affective or anxiety disorders, 24% with intermittent explosive disorders, and none with pyromania. Only 3.4% were diagnosed with ASPD. First-offense arsonists were more often psychotic than were recidivists. In addition, arsonists with a history of other crimes were diagnosed with pyromania in 24% of cases. They were also less likely to have schizophrenia, more likely to have a diagnosis of ASPD, and more likely to have been drinking when they set a fire.

Prison and Jail Samples

Hodgins and Cote (1993) assessed a random sample of 456 prison inmates using the Diagnostic Interview Schedule (DIS). One hundred and seven inmates received a diagnosis of an MMD, and 71 of those also received a diagnosis of ASPD. Offenders with mental disorders and with ASPD had significantly more convictions for nonviolent offenses, but approximately equal numbers of convictions for violent offenses. Cote and Hodgins (1990) also reported that 63% of prison inmates with schizophrenia also met criteria for ASPD. These data have important implications for diagnosis and treatment in a prison population: treatment of MMD may reduce crime associated with it but will have no effect on crime associated with ASPD. Prisoners should be assessed for both MMD and ASPD.

Cote and Hodgins (1992) compared the diagnoses of 87 prisoners convicted of homicide with the diagnoses of other prisoners. Thirty-five percent of the killers were diagnosed with MMD. This sample excluded killers who had committed suicide or who had been found incompetent to stand trial or not guilty by reason of insanity, so that these results substantially underestimate the association of MMD and homicide. The killers with MMD were significantly more often diagnosed with schizophrenia and with major depression associated with alcohol abuse or dependence than were control subjects. In 82% of cases, the MMD preceded the killing.

Rice and Harris (1995) studied 587 offenders with mental disorders who were confined in a maximum security psychiatric hospital. More than 80% of the men had been convicted of violent offenses. The authors studied psychiatric diagnosis in relation to violent recidivism among discharged patients. Principal diagnoses were DSM-III-R (American Psychiatric Association 1987) schizophrenia, psychopathy diagnosed according to Hare's Psychopathy Checklist—Revised (PCL-R), and alcohol abuse.

Almost no overlap occurred between schizophrenia and psychopathy in this population: Only 13 of 161 offenders with schizophrenia were also diagnosed as psychopathic. Men with schizophrenia in this selected population were less likely than others to recidivate (16% vs. 35%). However, 26% of men with schizophrenia and alcohol abuse were violent compared with 7% of men with schizophrenia without alcohol problems. The index offense was coded as "response to a delusion" in 112 cases (74 with schizophrenia), and these 112 men were less likely than other discharged patients to recidivate. The authors speculated that the reason for less violent recidivism among the patients with schizophrenia than among the control subjects was related to tighter community supervision and treatment of the patients with schizophrenia, but there were no data to support this.

A 1995 follow-up study compared released Canadian Federal prisoners with a psychotic diagnosis with a nonpsychotic control group (Porporino and Motiuk 1995). The psychotic patients received greater community supervision than the control subjects, and their parole was more often revoked, usually for failure to follow required treatment programs rather than for reoffending. More of those in the group without disorders than those in the group with disorders committed violent offenses while under supervision. These results at least suggested that the increased supervision of the group with mental disorders was successful in reducing recidivism.

In a study of 1,265 Canadian patients with schizophrenia remanded to a forensic hospital for competency to stand trial, 50%

were returned to court with no recommendation for further treatment (Smith et al. 1994). The authors concluded that inpatient competency evaluations are a waste of time and money. The 17 years of experience of one of us (JCB) with outpatient competency evaluations supports this conclusion.

Andersen et al. (1996) studied 228 randomly selected prisoners held for trial (i.e., on remand) in a Danish prison. All participants were given a psychiatric evaluation (Present State Examination), ICD-10 diagnoses, a PCL-R, and a global assessment. Diagnoses included 8% schizophrenia spectrum disorders, 11% affective disorders, 18% minor mental disorders, and 53% substance abuse disorders. Sixty-six individuals had several diagnoses; substance abuse was comorbid in 61 cases, ASPD in 26 cases. The authors noted that, "According to the *European Prison Rules* (citation omitted) . . . no psychotic subject should be in prison" (p. 71). As far as we are aware, there is no comparable set of rules in the United States, and it is a sad commentary that we have no similar statement of an ideal standard and that many psychotic persons are imprisoned here.

Teplin (1994) studied men awaiting trial in a Chicago jail. She found that 14% currently had an MMD, and another 29% had current drug or alcohol diagnoses. She compared the proportion of violent and nonviolent felonies between different diagnostic groups, including a group with no diagnosed disorder, and found that 12% to 15% of men with schizophrenia, major depression, and alcohol abuse/dependence had been arrested for a violent felony—not significantly different from men with no diagnosis. Men charged with drug offenses had significantly fewer violent felony charges than men with no diagnoses.

Teplin (1996) also studied 1,272 women awaiting trial in the same jail. She found that 34.5% of 38 women with schizophrenia had been charged with violent felonies. The range of violent felonies among other diagnostic groups was between 8.7% for drug abuse and 16.9% for major depression. Among the 540 women in the sample with no diagnosed disorder, 10.5% were charged with violent felonies. Although she did not find this latter comparison to be significant, recalculation suggests that it is (χ^2 with Yates' correction = 16.51, df = 1, $P < .001$).

Zapf et al. (1996) obtained interview and record review data from 790 male pretrial jail detainees in Vancouver, British Columbia, and compared homeless with domiciled men in this sample. Eight percent of the sample ($n = 53$) were homeless. Roughly 26% of both homeless and other defendants committed violent offenses. The homeless were more often mentally ill (36% vs. 17%) and showed more negative symptoms on the Brief Psychiatric Rating Scale. The differences between the New York (see the earlier discussion) and Vancouver data highlight the importance of considering social context when evaluating the relationship of mental disorder and crime. The homeless mentally ill in New York were far more often violent than those in Vancouver.

Persons With Mental Disorder

Case Register Study

The Maudsley Hospital, Britain's preeminent academic psychiatric institution, serves Camberwell, a working class area of London. Maudsley researchers established a case register of all patients served. Wessely et al. (1994) identified all those patients seen between 1965 and 1984 who received an ICD-9 diagnosis of schizophrenia, including schizoaffective, paraphrenia, and other nonorganic psychosis ($n = 538$). Control cases ($n = 538$) were patients without schizophrenia selected from the case register by matching each patient with schizophrenia for age ($\pm$ 5 years), gender, and date of service. The researchers rediagnosed all patients with schizophrenia using DSM-III-R criteria for schizophrenia. Results were generally similar for ICD-9 and DSM-III-R diagnostic analyses. Time at risk for criminal conviction was calculated for each subject by subtracting time in institutions from follow-up time.

Overall rates of conviction did not differ for patients with schizophrenia and control male patients, but men with schizophrenia had three times as many convictions for assault and other serious violence as the control men. Overall rates of conviction were higher for women with schizophrenia than for control subjects, as were rates of violent conviction. Rates of conviction for control subjects were no different or only slightly different from rates of conviction for England as a whole, and no different from those for a sample of nonpatients fortuitously studied from the Camberwell area. The authors did not report actual rates of violent crime. One limitation of this study is that it deals only with convictions, not with crimes for which there was no conviction. However, the study design controlled for gender, age, and date of first psychiatric service so that secular trends would affect patients with schizophrenia and control patients equally.

Inpatient Samples

Lindquist and Allebeck (1990) studied all ICD-9 patients diagnosed with schizophrenia from Stockholm who were born between 1920 and 1959 and who were alive in 1985 ($n = 644$). Forty-three schizophrenic patients committed violent crimes: 20 against life and health, 8 against liberty and peace, and 15 against public order. These were 3.9 times the expected number of violent crimes and 2.7 times the expected number of crimes against life and peace. The most serious crime was aggravated assault.

Modestin and Ammann (1995) studied a sample of all psychiatric inpatients hospitalized in 1987 in Berne, Switzerland, and a comparison group from the local population controlled for age, gender, marital status, social status, and size of community in which the person resided. "The importance of matching criteria was confirmed by the finding of a high proportion of control subjects with criminal records (36% of males and 6% of females) in comparison with the entire population of the Canton (15% of males and 2% of females)" (p. 670). Had the authors not matched or otherwise controlled for these variables, they would have reported spuriously large differences between patients and the population as a whole.

The male patients sampled, but not the female patients, had a higher proportion of conviction for violent crimes than did the control subjects. Presence of alcohol or drug abuse increased the risk of conviction, as did diagnosis of a concomitant personality disorder. Examining individual diagnoses, the authors note that patients with schizophrenia were not significantly more often convicted of violent crimes than control subjects. Although true, this observation is somewhat misleading in that 4% of patients with schizophrenia versus 1% of control subjects were convicted of violent offenses, an OR equal to 3.09. The result was insignificant only because the numbers were small. Similar but significant results were obtained for patients with affective disorders. If these two groups are combined as an MMD, the OR for violent convictions is 4.53 compared with control subjects ($P < .004$, two tailed).

The limitations of this study are, first, that the patients had all been hospitalized and, second, that the authors made no correction for the fact that chronic patients had somewhat less opportunity for conviction because they spent significant periods of time in hospital. This latter fact would bias the results toward an underestimate of the extent to which mental disorder and violent crime are related.

In a 1996 paper, Modestin and Ammann focused on all the patients with schizophrenia hospitalized in a 3-year period ($n = 282$). Compared with control subjects matched as above, these patients were five times more likely to have been convicted of violent crimes. Again, it is noteworthy that 34% of patients and 36% of control subjects had criminal records compared with 15% of the general male population. These studies and the Stockholm study are almost as compelling as the case register study because, as the authors noted, almost all patients with schizophrenia received hospital treatment at some point in their lives.

Volavka et al. (1995) did a retrospective record review and identified all patients in two New York hospitals arrested for a crime committed during hospitalization. These 73 were compared with 1,438 who were not arrested. Seventy-nine percent of arrests were for violent crimes. Axis I diagnoses, mostly schizophrenia, schizoaffective disorder, and bipolar disorder, did not differentiate arrestees from control subjects. However, 90% of arrestees had a diagnosis of substance abuse and/or personality disorder, usually ASPD. Patients arrested were more often young, African American, and male.

Grossman et al. (1995) studied the criminal histories of 172 patients with MMD at state hospitals in Illinois. Of the 172, 27% had committed violent crimes. In descending order, violence was associated with diagnoses of schizoaffective (40%), schizophrenic (28%), bipolar (24%), and unipolar (12.5%) disorders. Patients who were actively psychotic according to record review were more likely to have had a history of violent crime than other patients. Men and nonwhites were more likely to have had a history of violent crime, independent of diagnosis.

Lelliott et al. (1994) reported on a national survey of patients hospitalized in the United Kingdom for at least 6 months, but not more than 3 years. Hospital psychiatrists sent the authors data on 905 patients: 59% of the patients had schizophrenia, 18% had affective psychosis, and the rest had other diagnoses. Roughly one-third had a second diagnosis, but only 5% of patients had diagnoses of alcohol or drug dependence. About 30% had a history of dangerousness or criminality, 18% had committed a serious act of violence, 11% had shown other dangerous or criminal behavior. Youth and male gender were associated with a history of serious violence. No data on diagnosis and serious violence were reported. Twenty-nine percent of the sample had been formally detained, that is, admitted after a criminal proceeding, as contrasted with 9% of a similar sample 20 years earlier. This study illustrates that in the United Kingdom, as in the United States, young, chronically ill mental patients are violent far more often than was true 20 years ago. The low percentage of substance abuse contrasts markedly with that in the United States.

Rasmussen and Levander (1996) studied 94 patients referred to the maximum security hospital in Norway. Seventy percent came from hospitals; 30% came from prisons. Almost half of the patients were under preventive detention. The authors examined comorbidity and found that 12 of 48 patients with DSM-III-R schizophrenia were also psychopathic (PCL-R > 30). These data from "the most violent and unmanageable mentally ill individuals in a population of 4 million people" contradict the belief that ASPD and schizophrenia are seldom found together.

Shah et al. (1994) compared 62 patients hospitalized as not guilty by reason of insanity (NGRI) with 62 hospitalized control subjects. The NGRI sample were more often diagnosed with paranoid schizophrenia, had been hospitalized significantly longer than control subjects, and were rated as better behaviorally adjusted than control subjects. The authors speculated that these homicidal (40%) and aggravated assaulting (31%) patients were better adjusted because patients with paranoid schizophrenia often improved more with treatment than patients with other types of schizophrenia, and because judges were reluctant to let these seriously violent patients out of the hospital, even when they were much improved.

Seig et al. (1995) compared 37 women with 112 men found NGRI in Colorado. More women than men had killed (43% vs. 19%) or attempted to kill (11% vs. 0%), but men had more often sexually assaulted (18% vs. 0%). More women than men had a history of suicide attempt before the index crime (49% vs. 30%). Women were more often diagnosed with mood disorders and borderline personality disorder than were men. Men were more often diagnosed with substance abuse/dependence (63% vs. 16%).

Lundy et al. (1993) obtained criminal records for 170 adults who had been hospitalized as children (average age at discharge was 9.6 years). Twenty-three men, but none of the women, had been to prison—10 for violent crimes. Seven of these 10 were diagnosed with ASPD.

Outpatient Samples

Asnis et al. (1994) reported on a detailed self-report questionnaire on homicidal ideation and attempts that 517 outpatients completed. Twenty-two patients (4%) reported homicidal attempts. The noteworthy result was that 21 of these 22 had attempted suicide, but homicidal ideation was not related to attempted suicide.

Violence in Response to Delusions

Taylor (1985) initially reported the association between delusions and violent offending, and one of us (JCB) has unpublished data supporting this association as well. It is important to investigate further what distinguishes patients who act on delusions from those who do not, because some of those who act do act violently. Wessely et al. (1993) and Buchanan et al. (1993) have studied this problem.

These investigators (Wessely et al. 1993; Buchanan et al. 1993) studied consecutive patients with functional psychoses admitted to several London hospitals ($n = 83$). Patients and family were interviewed and the authors completed the Maudsley Assessment of Delusions (MADS) scale for each patient. This scale describes variables related to patient delusions, such as content, certainty, preoccupation, systematization, and emotional response. The authors refer to these variables as the phenomenology of delusions.

Sixty percent of patients had taken action in response to delusions—for example, written to someone, tried to get something they believed was happening to stop, or tried to protect themselves, or to escape; 18% had hit someone; 14% had harmed themselves; and 19% had broken something. Breaking something was associated with self-reports of delusions of catastrophe, but not with paranoid delusions.

According to relatives, 19 of these patients had been violent before admission, 2 seriously. Family reports linked delusions of persecution with patient action, but patients whom relatives reported as having delusions of catastrophe were less likely to act on them than other patients—a finding opposite to the patient report data.

When patients described their behavior, there was an association between looking and finding evidence to support the delusion and acting on it. Patients who were sad or frightened by their delusions were more likely to act on them than others. Family reports did not relate to the phenomenology of patient delusions. This careful, initial study raises important questions about why relatives' reports are so different from those of patients. Junginger (1996) also has reviewed the literature on the relationship between violence, psychosis, and characteristics of delusions, arguing for the importance of further studies, such as the two reviewed earlier.

Genesis of Violent Behavior in Persons With Axis I Psychopathology

Brain Dysfunction

Results of numerous neuropsychological studies conducted over the past 20 years suggest that a relationship exists between neuropsychological dysfunction and criminality and between poor neuropsychological test performance and Axis I disorders (e.g., psychosis, depression, posttraumatic stress disorder, attention-deficit/hyperactivity disorder, learning disorders). However, few studies have been explicitly designed to test whether the populations having both Axis I disorders and violent criminal behavior are more impaired as determined by neuropsychological tests than appropriate control groups.

Adams et al. (1990) administered the Luria-Nebraska Battery to 37 patients with schizophrenia in a jail-inpatient unit. All but 5 had histories of violent crime. Impairment, as determined by the Luria, and severity of violent crime were related, and the 5 most violent patients were all impaired according to the Luria results.

Nestor (1992) reviewed neuropsychological testing in 40 inpatients at a maximum security psychiatric facility. Twenty-eight of the 40 had killed; the other 12 had committed other violent crimes. Nestor compared 22 men who committed their crime at mean age 19.3 with a group who committed their crime at a mean age of 41.4. The groups were tested at mean ages of 20.2 and 46.4, respectively. Fourteen men in each group had killed. Younger patients exhibited significantly higher rates of both learning disability and history of childhood conduct disorder, and more than twice as many prior arrests (64 vs. 28). More men in the older group were psychotic when tested, an average of 40 days after the criminal act. The older men who killed were significantly more likely to have acted alone and to have killed a significant other.

Raine et al. (1994b) compared 22 individuals who were found NGRI for murder with 22 matched control subjects. Analyzing positron-emission tomography (PET) scan data obtained during continuous performance testing, the authors found lower glucose metabolism in the lateral and medial prefrontal cortex of the NGRI sample as compared with control subjects. Other brain regions did not differ. The authors suggested that serious violence may be related to prefrontal cortical deficits.

Wong et al. (1994) reported on extensive neurological and neuropsychological evaluation of 372 male patients at Broadmoor, a maximum security forensic hospital. Patients were divided into three groups from least to most violent. Roughly 70% of all patients had Axis I diagnoses, and roughly 25% of the two more violent groups had ASPD. The three groups did not differ in IQ or in generalized electroencephalogram (EEG) abnormalities. Increasing violence was associated with increased likelihood of abnormal temporal lobe EEG findings, from 2.4% to 3.4% to 20% across the three groups. Computerized tomography (CT) findings were similarly abnormal. Percentages of abnormal focal temporal abnormalities on CT went from 6.7% to 7.5% to 41% across the three groups. The authors concluded that these localized findings may relate specifically to violence rather than to head injury or mental illness.

Low Socioeconomic Status

Hiday (1995) argued vigorously that certain social conditions predisposed to violence and mental disorder. For example, members of a persecuted minority or victimized underclass may develop paranoid fearfulness. Persons with MMD may live in a violent subculture, and their own irritability may lead to confrontations that become violent. She asserted that it was simplistic to ignore the role of social context in trying to understand how mental state and behavior are related. She also argued for the importance of assessing comorbid substance abuse and ASPD when studying MMD and violent crime. This view was reinforced by the review of Link and Stueve (1995).

Dohrenwend et al. (1992) have written an important paper on socioeconomic status and psychiatric disorders. Although not about violent crime and mental disorder per se, it provided important context for thinking about the relationship of socioeconomic status and ethnicity as these may relate to violent crime committed by persons with mental disorders. The authors tested two competing theories of the relationship between social class and mental disorders. Social causation theory predicts that frustration experienced by the disadvantaged group at every class level leads to higher rates of mental disorder than for the advantaged group. Social selection theory predicts that an intergenerational process of sorting and selection goes on such that the able rise and the disabled sink, so that at each class level the advantaged group has higher rates of mental disorders.

By studying North African Jews in Israel who are a disadvantaged group, as compared with Israeli Jews of European origin, the authors were able to separate the effects of race/ethnicity and class membership. The data supported a social selection effect for schizophrenia, and a social causation effect for depression in women and for ASPD and substance abuse in men.

Biological and Social Risk Factor Interactions

An initial study by Raine et al. (1994a) showed that 4.4% of all live male births in a Danish cohort resulted in infants who experienced birth complications and maternal rejection in the first year of life. At age 18, these men accounted for 18% of all violent crimes in the sample.

In a later study, the authors studied 423 of the original cohort more intensively (Raine et al. 1996). They collected prospective data on pregnancy and birth complications, neonatal maturity, neurological status in the first week of life, and motor development at 1 year of age. Psychosocial data were obtained in an interview with the mothers when the young men were age 17 to 19. Violent crime was defined as arrests for murder or attempted murder, assault, rape, robbery, illegal possession of a weapon, or threats of violence. Criminal status was assessed from a national register when the men in the sample were 20 to 22 years old.

Cluster analysis generated three groups. The biosocial group ($n = 176$) had neurological problems in the first week of life and social risk factors for crime—maternal rejection, family conflict or instability, or a criminal parent. The biological group ($n = 106$) had biological deficits only: pregnancy and birth complications, prematurity, and slow motor development. The social group ($n = 115$) grew up in poverty with more negative social, economic, educational, employment, and living situations. They grew up in poverty, but not necessarily in bad homes. In fact, they had significantly earlier motor development, and they experienced less parental discord. A normal control group was defined as those individuals who had neither biological nor social deficits.

The biosocial group committed 70% of all the crimes committed. They committed 2.3 times as much violent crime as the other two subject groups, and more of them committed violent crime than did normal control subjects (12.6% vs. 2.3%). The authors commented that much crime could be prevented by early intervention in the group at biological risk, or by addressing some psychosocial risk factors, for example by educating young adolescents on parenting, family planning, and conflict management.

In their most recent report (Raine et al. 1997), the authors reported on the follow-up of this sample to age 34. There was an interaction between maternal rejection (defined as either a maternal attempt to abort or institutional placement during the first year of life) and being raised in poor social circumstances (unmarried mother, low socioeconomic status, poor home conditions, young mother, or unwanted pregnancy) with early-onset violent crime (robbery, rape, or murder before age 18), but not with later-onset violent crime (over age 18). These findings were independent of maternal mental disorder.

Summary and Conclusions

This review illustrates that the study of mental disorder and violent crime is extraordinarily active and vigorous. It is now a well-established fact that schizophrenia increases the risk of homicide and other violent crime. It is striking that work done in many different countries has resulted in remarkably similar findings. A smaller number of studies documents a relationship between MMD generally and violent crime.

Unfortunately, the fact that people with schizophrenia are more likely to commit criminal violence than other people can lead to further scapegoating of the mentally ill and to further efforts to marginalize them. In interpreting these results, therefore, it is important to keep the following in mind:

- The vast majority of persons with MMD do not commit violent crimes.
- When persons with MDD do commit violent crimes, they usually do so against family members and significant others, not against strangers. The media myth of the violent schizophrenic patient lashing out randomly against strangers is rarely confirmed in reality.
- With appropriate treatment, the likelihood that a person with MMD will commit a violent crime can be greatly reduced. It is a fair inference that people with schizophrenia who are compliant with a treatment regimen are at no greater risk of violence than anyone else. Or, if there is an increased risk, the increase is so small as to be trivial.
- The real public health issue concerning mental disorder and violence is alcohol abuse. Much of the violent crime in the United States occurs under the influence of alcohol. Professional attention or the attention of policymakers should not be diverted from this fact by the findings reported in this chapter.

It is important to remember that the base rates of mental disorder are similar in many of the countries reporting the relationship of schizophrenia and homicide. However, the base rate of homicide in many of these countries is 10% of that in the United States. Americans are more accepting of social conditions that increase the risk of homicide—gun-owning citizenry for example—so that in the United States there are proportionately more homicides committed by people without MMD. In the United Kingdom, almost all homicide defendants receive a forensic psychiatric evaluation on the theory that someone who commits a homicide is likely to have an MMD. In this country, there is less reason to believe that homicide may imply an MMD, including schizophrenia.

Several studies note a greatly increased risk of violent crime among patients with schizophrenia who abuse alcohol. We found no paper that addressed the question of whether this effect is additive or whether there is also an interaction that increased the risk of violent crime even further. This is an important topic for future research. Studies that report the comorbidity of schizophrenia and ASPD report widely varying proportions—from approximately 8% (Rice and Harris 1995) or 10% (Repo et al. 1997) to 63% (Cote and Hodgins 1990). The reasons for this are also unclear and deserve research attention.

Several authors find that the relationship between schizophrenia or MMD and homicide or violent crime is stronger for women than for men. This is consistent with studies that have found that female patients are more often violent than male patients (e.g., Beck et al. 1991).

This review also illustrates the importance of social context. The widely varying numbers of stranger victims in Milwaukee and New York, and the differences in crime committed by homeless mentally ill in Vancouver and New York point to the importance of social context variables in the genesis of violence among persons with mental illness. The number of studies we reviewed that carefully controlled social variables and still found differences in rates of violent crime between schizophrenic patients and others, argues strongly that these relationships are primary. They are unlikely to be functions of some third unrecognized and unmeasured variable.

The large numbers of people with mental disorders among

pretrial jail inmates is a source of concern, especially in the light of the European Prison Rules against imprisoning psychotic persons. The criminally mentally ill are probably among the most underserved populations in America with regard to their mental health care.

The work on delusions and violent behavior—behavior that would be considered crime if it were officially recognized—is only just beginning. The effort to characterize delusions and to discover what distinguishes delusional patients who are violent from those who are not is an important contemporary area of study.

We found few brain imaging studies of persons with Axis I mental disorder who had committed violent crimes. One pointed to temporal abnormalities, the other to frontal abnormalities. Clearly, this is a research area that will grow.

The work on pregnancy and birth complications interacting with poor upbringing to produce violent criminality appears to be a critically important finding. If at all possible, this line of investigation should be pursued in the United States, with the aim of replicating findings suggesting crucial biological and social risk factor interactions in the genesis of violent behavior in persons with Axis I psychopathology.

References

Adams JJ, Meloy JR, Moritz MS: Neuropsychological deficits and violent behavior in incarcerated schizophrenics. J Nerv Ment Dis 178:253–256, 1990

American Psychiatric Association: Diagnostic and Statistical Manual of Mental Disorders, 3rd Edition, Revised. Washington, DC, American Psychiatric Association, 1987

Andersen HS, Sestoft D, Lillebaek T, et al: Prevalence of ICD-10 psychiatric morbidity in random samples of prisoners on remand. Int J Law Psychiatry 19:61–74, 1996

Asnis GM, Kaplan ML, van Prang HM, et al: Homicidal behaviors among psychiatric outpatients. Hosp Community Psychiatry 45:127–132, 1994

Beck JC, White KA, Gage B: Emergency psychiatric assessment of violence. Am J Psychiatry 148:1562–1565, 1991

Buchanan A, Reed A, Wessely S, et al: Acting on delusions, II: the phenomenological correlates of acting on delusions. Br J Psychiatry 163:77–81, 1993

Cote G, Hodgins S: Co-occurring mental disorders among criminal offenders. Bull Am Acad Psychiatry Law 18:271–281, 1990

Cote G, Hodgins S: The prevalence of major mental disorders among homicide offenders. Int J Law Psychiatry 15:89–99, 1992

Dohrenwend BP, Levav I, Shrout PE, et al: Socioeconomic status and psychiatric disorders: the causation-selection issue. Science 255:946–951, 1992

Eronen M, Hakola P, Tiihonen J: Mental disorders and homicidal behavior in Finland. Arch Gen Psychiatry 53:497–501, 1996a

Eronen M, Tiihonen J, Hakola P: Schizophrenia and homicidal behavior. Schizophr Bull 22:83–89, 1996b

Eronen M, Hakola P, Tiihonen J: Factors associated with homicide recidivism in a 13-year sample of homicide offenders in Finland. Psychiatric Services 47:403–406, 1996c

Euripides: Herakles, in Complete Greek Tragedies, Vol 3. Edited by Green D, Lattimore R. Chicago, IL, University of Chicago Press, 1959, pp 283–339

Grossman LS, Haywood TW, Cavanaugh JL, et al: State psychiatric hospital patients with past arrests for violent crimes. Psychiatr Serv 46:790–795, 1995

Hiday VA: The social context of mental illness and violence. J Health Soc Behav 36:122–137, 1995

Hodgins S, Cote G: Major mental disorder and antisocial personality disorder: a criminal combination. Bull Am Acad Psychiatry Law 21:155–160, 1993

Hodgins S, Mednick SA, Brennan PA, et al: Mental disorder and crime. Arch Gen Psychiatry 53:489–496, 1996

Jones v United States, U.S. S.Ct. 463, 354 (1983)

Junginger J: Psychosis and violence: the case for a content analysis of psychotic experience. Schizophr Bull 22:91–103, 1996

Lelliott P, Wing J, Clifford P: A national audit of new long-stay psychiatric patients, I: method and description of the cohort. Br J Psychiatry 165:160–169, 1994

Lindquist P, Allebeck P: Schizophrenia and violent crime. Br J Psychiatry 157:345–350, 1990

Link BG, Steuve A: Psychotic symptoms and the violent/illegal behavior of mental patients compared to community controls, in Violence and Mental Disorder. Edited by Monahan J, Steadman HJ. Chicago, IL, University of Chicago Press, 1994, pp 137–160

Link BG, Stueve A: Evidence bearing on mental illness as a possible cause of violent behavior. Epidemiol Rev 17:172–181, 1995

Link BG, Cullen F, Andrews H: Violent and illegal behavior of current and former mental patients compared to community controls. Am Soc Rev 57:272–292, 1992

Lundy MG, Pfohl BM, Kuperman S: Adult criminality among formerly hospitalized child psychiatric patients. J Am Acad Child Adolesc Psychiatry 32:568–576, 1993

Malmquist C: Depression and homicidal violence. Int J Law Psychiatry 18:145–162, 1995

Martell DA, Rosner R, Harmon RB: Base-rate estimates of criminal behavior by homeless mentally ill persons in New York City. Psychiatr Serv 46:596–600, 1995

Modestin J, Ammann R: Mental disorder and criminal behaviour. Br J Psychiatry 166:667–675, 1995

Modestin J, Ammann R: Mental disorder and criminality: male schizophrenia. Schizophr Bull 22:69–82, 1996

Monahan J, Steadman HJ: Crime and Mental Disorder. Washington, DC: National Institute of Justice, research in brief, September, 1984

Najera v Southern Pacific Co., 191 Cal App2d 634, 649 (1961)

Nestor PG: Neuropsychological and clinical correlates of murder and other forms of extreme violence in a forensic psychiatric population. J Nerv Ment Dis 180:418–423, 1992

Porporino FJ, Motiuk LL: The prison careers of mentally disordered offenders. Int J Law Psychiatry 18:29–44, 1995

Raine A, Brennan P, Mednick SA: Birth complications combined with early maternal rejection at age 1 year predispose to violent crime at age 18 years. Arch Gen Psychiatry 51:984–988, 1994a

Raine A, Buchsbaum MS, Stanley J, et al: Selective reductions in prefrontal glucose metabolism in murderers. Biol Psychiatry 36:365–373, 1994b

Raine A, Brennan P, Mednick B, et al: High rates of violence, crime, academic problems, and behavioral problems in males with both early neuromotor deficits and unstable family environments. Arch Gen Psychiatry 53:544–549, 1996

Raine A, Brennan P, Mednick SA: Interaction between birth complications and early maternal rejection in predisposing individuals to adult violence: specificity to serious, early-onset violence. Am J Psychiatry 154:1265–1271, 1997

Rasmussen K, Levander S: Symptoms and personality characteristics of patients in a maximum security psychiatric unit. Int J Law Psychiatry 19:27–37, 1996

Repo E, Vikkunen M, Rawlings R, et al: Criminal and psychiatric histories of Finnish arsonists. Acta Psychiatr Scand 95:318–323, 1997

Rice ME, Harris GT: Psychopathy, schizophrenia, alcohol abuse, and violent recidivism. Int J Law Psychiatry 18:333–342, 1995

Seig A, Ball E, Menninger JA: A comparison of female versus male insanity acquittees in Colorado. Bull Am Acad Psychiatry Law 23:523–532, 1995

Shah PJ, Greenberg WM, Convit A: Hospitalized insanity acquittees' level of functioning. Bull Am Acad Psychiatry Law 22:85–93, 1994

Signorelli N: The stigma of mental illness on television. J Broadcasting Electronic Media 33:325–331, 1989

Smith J, Hucker S: Schizophrenia and substance abuse. Br J Psychiatry 165:13–21, 1994b

Smith J, Grant F, Brinded P: Schizophrenics remanded to the forensic psychiatric institute of British Columbia, 1975–1990. Med Sci Law 34:221–226, 1994

Steury EH, Choinski M: "Normal" crimes and mental disorder: a two-group comparison of deadly and dangerous felonies. Int J Law Psychiatry 18:183–207, 1995

Swanson JW: Mental disorder, substance abuse and community violence: an epidemiologic approach, in Violence and Mental Disorder. Edited by Monahan J, Steadman HJ. Chicago, IL, University of Chicago Press, 1994, pp 101–136

Swanson JW, Holzer CE, Ganju VK, et al: Violence and psychiatric disorder in the community: evidence from the epidemiologic catchment area surveys. Hosp Community Psychiatry 41:761–770, 1990

Taylor PJ: Motives for offending among violent and psychotic men. Br J Psychiatry 147:491–498, 1985

Teplin LA: Psychiatric and substance abuse disorders among male urban jail detainees. Am J Public Health 84:290–293, 1994

Teplin LA: Prevalence of psychiatric disorders among incarcerated women, I: pretrial jail detainees. Arch Gen Psychiatry 43:505–511, 1996

Tiihonen J: Criminality associated with mental disorders and intellectual deficiency. Arch Gen Psychiatry 50:917–918, 1993

Tiihonen J, Hakola P, Eronen M: Risk of homicidal behavior among discharged forensic psychiatric patients. Forensic Sci Int 79:123–129, 1996

Volavka J, Mohammad Y, Vitrai J, et al: Characteristics of state hospital patients arrested for offenses committed during hospitalization. Psychiatr Serv 46:796–800, 1995

Wessely S, Buchanan A, Reed J, et al: Acting on delusions, I: prevalence. Br J Psychiatry 163:69–76, 1993

Wessely SC, Castle D, Douglas AJ, et al: The criminal careers of incident cases of schizophrenia. Psychol Med 24:483–502, 1994

Widom CS, Maxfield MG: A prospective examination of risk for violence among abused and neglected children. Ann NY Acad Sci 794:224–237, 1996

Wong MTH, Lumsden J, Fenton GW, et al: Electroencephalography, computed tomography and violence ratings of male patients in a maximum-security mental hospital. Acta Psychiatr Scand 90:97–101, 1994

Zapf PA, Roesch R, Hart SD: An examination of the relationship of homelessness to mental disorder, criminal behaviour, and health care in a pretrial jail population. Can J Psychiatry 41:435–440, 1996

Chapter 2

The Personalities of Murderers: The Importance of Psychopathy and Sadism

Michael H. Stone, M.D.

Few studies in the forensic literature have been devoted to the personality profiles of offenders committing unlawful homicide (i.e., murder—as opposed to killing in self-defense, which is lawful homicide). Those articles that do touch on personality concentrate either on incarcerated offenders in prisons or in forensic psychiatric hospitals, or else on offenders with a limited array of personality disturbances, such as antisocial personality disorder (ASPD) (as defined by DSM-III [American Psychiatric Association 1980]/DSM-IV [American Psychiatric Association 1994]), or psychopathy (as defined by Robert Hare and his colleagues: Hare 1996; Hare et al. 1990). Only a few articles focus solely on persons who have murdered.

Ultimately, one wants to be able to answer such questions as the following:

- How commonly will one see personality disorders in a population of murderers, and what are the most prevalent types?
- Are there personality profiles that correlate strongly with particular types of homicide?
- Perhaps most important, are there profiles that best predict the propensity to commit homicide in the future (or—in the case of incarcerated murderers—to kill again if released)?

Murder is a broad umbrella under which many subtypes are found—making generalizations about personality factors hazardous. Cultural differences play a role also: The murder rate is considerably higher in the United States (9 to 10 per 100,000 per year) compared with many countries in Western Europe (1 per 100,000 per year) or Japan (0.3 per 100,000 per year) (Wolfgang 1986). Serial sexual homicide—a topic that has engendered fascination in recent years—is all but unknown in Spain, Italy, and Japan, yet considerably more common (though still mercifully rare, statistically speaking) in America.

Biographies as Source Material About Personality

It is difficult even for forensic psychiatrists to accumulate detailed information, obtained from direct interview, about the personality profiles of murderers in a large enough sample of individuals to permit statistical analysis. Full-length biographies can supplement fairly adequately the otherwise limited data set derived from clinical experience. For much of the following material I have relied on my reading of nearly 300 such biographies of murderers. Most of these books provide rich material concerning personality traits of the murderers in question, as provided by their relatives, acquaintances, and surviving victims, as well as by law enforcement personnel, attorneys, and mental health professionals involved in their cases. From this biographical material I have been able to construct a computerized database composed of many variables, including those relating to DSM descriptors of personality disorders. This material constitutes the "series" I refer to in many of the following remarks. Admittedly, this biographical series is not representative of murders in the United States in general. Only 1 murderer out of about 1,100 becomes the subject of a full-length book. These books center necessarily on dramatic cases—where the crime was 1) particularly gruesome, 2) unusually hard to solve, or 3) involved a person whom one would not ordinarily think likely to murder. As a result, there are no books devoted to barroom brawl murders, drug deals gone bad, and the like. Instead, the biographies concentrate on persons committing serial murder (especially, serial sexual homicide), spousal murder within affluent families, and the murder of relatives for financial gain. Serial killers are so common a subject for full-length biographies that the (in my series, 77) books devoted to this topic actually are representative of the group as a whole.

Antisociality Among Persons Who Murder

Murder, along with torture, stands at the summit of antisocial acts—yet not all murderers show antisocial personality as defined by DSM-IV, let alone a high Psychopathy Checklist (PCL) (Hare et al. 1990) score. But there is no question that antisocial personality (including some of its semantic close cousins: sociopathy, psychopathy, dyssocial personality) is significantly overrepresented, compared with the general population, in any sample of offenders who commit homicide. In a Danish study by Andersen et al. (1996), for example, about one prisoner in six (whether incarcerated for murder or for other crimes, and whether in solitary or shared confinement) was diagnosed as a "dyssocial personality." In a Norwegian study, Rasmussen and Levander (1995) looked at the personality profiles of offenders remanded to a forensic psychiatric hospital because of concomitant mental illness. Eighty-seven of the 94 participants were male, and of the 87, a third were adjudged to have ASPD by DSM-III-R (American Psychiatric Association 1987) criteria (none of the 7 women did). Three of the men (3.5%) and 4 of the women (57%) showed borderline personality disorder (BPD). Fifteen of the men (and none of the women) were diagnosed "other personality disorder." In two-fifths of both gender groups no personality disorder was noted. In still another Scandinavian study, Eronen et al. (1996) were impressed by the degree to which mental illness heightened the risk for homicidal behavior. Given the diagnosis of schizophrenia, for example, the odds ratio (OR) of homicidal violence was increased 8-fold in men, 6.5-fold in women. Among those with ASPD (here considered as a "mental illness") the OR was higher by a factor of 10 in the males, by a factor of 50 in the females. No such increase was noted when the main diagnosis was affective or anxiety disorder. The Finnish group did not examine in extenso the personality profiles of the mentally ill who committed murder but did underline the correlation between ASPD and homicide.

In an extensive study of serial sexual homicide undertaken by Geberth and Turco (1997), the correlation between ASPD and homicide was invariably evident. All 68 of the "serial killers" about whom the authors had data sufficient to complete their protocols (from an original sample of 248 who had violated their victims sexually) met DSM-IV criteria for ASPD. Commenting on the areas of overlap and dysjunction between ASPD and homicide, Geberth stated: "Without doubt, not all those with antisocial personality will kill, and not all serial murderers are psychopaths" (p. 51). Although no one seriously questions the first clause in that statement, the correlation between serial homicide and psychopathy may be tighter than the authors are willing to concede. But this necessitates our looking more closely at the distinctions between "antisociality" (in the DSM usage) and "psychopathy," as the latter is currently defined.

Psychopathy as a Personality Type

The concept of psychopathy has evolved from a term whose etymology simply implies "illness of the mind," to the notion of "constitutionally inferior"—in the sense of being irresponsible and morally weak throughout life. Kraepelin used the phrase "psychopathic personality" to signify a general mental abnormality (1909–1915). Some of his examples concerned antisocial behavior, as when he spoke of *Zechprellerei* (leaving restaurants without paying), *Streitzucht* (quarrelsomeness), and *Reuelosigkeit* (lack of repentance), whereas his *Haltlosingkeit* (uninhibitedness) and *Verschrobenheit* (eccentricity) did not carry an overtone of amorality. "Psychopathy" as a term embodying the qualities of amorality and lack of remorse (noted in some of Kraepelin's examples)—coupled with manipulativeness, glibness, and chronic lying, *yet in the absence of psychosis*—was promulgated by Hervey

---

Cleckley in his masterful monograph, appearing first in 1941. In later editions Cleckley enumerated some 16 attributes common to this group of persons, who, as he put it, wore the "mask of sanity" (1972). In recent years the revision of this list worked out by Hare and his colleagues (Hare et al. 1990)—the *Revised Psychopathy Checklist* (PCL-R)—has gained wide popularity and is fast becoming a standard instrument in forensic psychiatry. The checklist now contains 20 items. Of these, 15 are true personality traits and include such attributes as glibness, grandiose sense of self-worth, pathological lying, conning (manipulativeness), callousness, impulsivity, and irresponsibility. The remainder are general items such as juvenile delinquency, revocation of conditional release (in the case of incarcerated offenders), and criminal versatility (meaning a propensity toward the commission of several different kinds of crime, such as theft, forgery, rape, and murder).

The 15 personality traits of the PCL-R make the Hare checklist more clearly oriented toward personality, in the strict sense of the word, than was the case with the definition of ASPD in DSM-III. There the emphasis was on objectifiable acts such as truancy, stealing, nonpayment of child support, and the like. The DSM-IV definition has approached the PCL-R in stressing personality features: Five of the seven items relate clearly to personality (deceitfulness, impulsivity, irritability/aggressiveness, irresponsibility, and lack of remorse). From a diagnostic standpoint, it is more difficult to confirm the presence of psychopathy in the Cleckley/Hare sense than the presence of antisocial personality as defined by DSM-III. DSM-IV occupies an intermediate position—though closer in spirit to the PCL-R. This, I believe, represents a salutary change. The traits of deceitfulness and conning are much more difficult to pin down in brief interviews with, or brief exposures to, psychopathic persons. They are, after all, highly adept at fooling others—including astute diagnosticians and law enforcement personnel. Yet traits of this sort go to the essence of what it is clinicians want to identify and distinguish, when assessing offenders and especially when making prognostic evaluations of the most violent offenders: those who have committed homicide or torture. There is enough importance in this task to warrant, when one is faced with the possibility of a psychopathic diagnosis, extensive interviews over time with the person in question, and interviews with other informants (e.g., relatives, acquaintances) who may have been cheated, duped, harmed, or otherwise adversely affected and who can supply the relevant information that the psychopath had been at pains to conceal.

Hare and his colleagues have shown that the PCL-R can be understood as the amalgam of two factors (Harpur et al. 1988). Factor 1 concerns the interpersonal aspects of psychopathy, especially those involving narcissistic traits. Included are *egocentricity, manipulativeness, callousness,* and *lack of remorse*. These are the "core" psychopathic qualities. Factor 2 relates to the impulsive, unstable, and irresponsible lifestyle characteristics of many psychopaths. Factor 1 correlates strongly with narcissistic personality disorder, with "Machiavellianism" (cunning and deceitfulness as noted not in Machiavelli himself, but in psychopaths and in the political tyrants Machiavelli was writing about), and (most important) with the predisposition to violence and recidivism. Rice and Harris (1995) noted, for example, that high PCL-R psychopathy scores were more highly correlated with recidivism in violent offenders than was alcoholism or schizophrenia. Similarly, Serin and Amos (1995) noted the close correlation between the PCL-R score (which can range from 0 to 40) and recidivism after release: Those with scores of 0–10 failed 3% of the time; offenders in the highest decile (31–40) failed in 33% of cases.

Factor 2, as Hare mentions (1996, p. 31), correlates with DSM ASPD, with criminal and antisocial behaviors, and with substance abuse. High Factor 2 scores are also found less often in those with high socioeconomic status, education, and IQ.

Given these distinctions, we would expect that, in a population of murderers, those who operate chiefly out of stealth, cunning, careful premeditation, and wanton disregard for the feelings of others, and who rely on outward charm to diminish the wariness of potential victims, would score high on Hare's

Factor 1. In contrast, those who kill on impulse, as in jealous rages, barroom brawls, heated family disputes, and the like, would score higher on Factor 2. Of course, persons with PCL-R scores in the high 30s necessarily exhibit intense degrees of both the narcissism and the impulsivity factors.

Though we will be paying closer attention to these factors when we look, later on, at the life stories and crime histories within the many subtypes of homicide, we can already appreciate how murderers who are psychopathic mainly with the Factor 1 characteristics would be found among serial killers, persons who hire "hit men" to kill a spouse, poisoners, and so on. Psychopaths who are mostly Factor 2 in typology would fill the ranks of rageful men who earn newspaper fame for a day or two by violating orders of restraint and killing wives or lovers, or inebriated men who on impulse kill indigent strangers sleeping in the street. Also of this Factor 2 type was the highly narcissistic and impulsive man (Andrew Cunanan) whose first two murder victims were killed out of jealousy, and whose fifth victim was the famous designer Gianni Versace (*New York Times*, July 16, 1997). The topic of narcissistic personality is in itself of great importance in any discussion of personality factors in murderers; thus, some comments on narcissism are in order here.

Narcissistic Personality in Murderers

A close correspondence exists between the Hare Factor 1 traits and the defining items of DSM-IV's narcissistic personality disorder (NPD). The latter mentions grandiose sense of self-importance, fantasies of unlimited success (really a variant of grandiosity), exploitativeness (similar to conning/manipulativeness), entitlement, lack of empathy (similar to callousness), and arrogance. In addition, persons with NPD are often driven by a sense of specialness and by envy.

Since one of the core features of both antisociality and psychopathy is egocentricity (specifically, adhering only to one's own rules while being contemptuous of the rules and needs of others), it would be no rash overstatement to assert that persons with ASPD or psychopathy also exhibit powerful narcissistic traits, if not full-blown, concomitant NPD. The reverse is of course not true: Many persons with NPD are neither antisocial nor psychopathic. Those who attempt or carry out murder, on the other hand, are in the vast majority of cases narcissistic— even more often, actually, than they would be diagnosed with ASPD or psychopathy. Exceptions might be instances when someone kills a tormentor, or persistent stalker, or in certain cases of vigilantism. An instance of the latter concerned the citizens of Skidmore, Missouri, who shot and killed Ken McElroy after years of his having raped, terrorized, stolen, and shot at various townspeople, while continually escaping punishment via clever defense attorneys (Maclean 1988).

In flamboyant murder cases that make the headlines or that inspire a book, one routinely encounters intense narcissistic and psychopathic traits. This is evident in cases of premeditated murder to gain inheritance or insurance, as well as in cases of serial sexual homicide. An example of murder to "accelerate" an inheritance is that of the celebrated Menendez brothers in Los Angeles (Dunne 1993), who killed both parents to enrich themselves (for which they were convicted in 1996). Another example concerns Dana Ewell (Smith 1997), a young man who promised a college friend half the $8 million he expected to inherit, if that friend would murder his parents and sister. Dana was described as grandiose, a pathological liar (boasting he had an IQ of 180 and that, while in college, he had become a "self-made" millionaire—as his father had actually been), obsessed with wealth, fussy, overbearing, egocentric, callous, arrogant, and contemptuous.

As I hope to document further on, narcissistic and antisocial/ psychopathic traits blend together to form a personality configuration that is so common as to be almost ubiquitous among murderers of almost every type. Certain other personality tendencies are less common within this domain, but of great importance, insofar as they predispose to several varieties of repetitive, grotesque, or especially savage murder. Here I refer to schizoid, paranoid, borderline, and sadistic traits.

Schizoid Personality in Relation to Murder

The salient features of schizoid personality disorder (DSM-IV) are aloofness, lack of close friends or confidants, and emotional coldness or detachment. As with many personality disorders, the disorder in question is often comorbid with others. This is especially true of borderline personality disorder (BPD), as shown by Oldham et al. (1992), but is common with schizoid persons also—many of whom (especially those encountered in the forensic literature) show paranoid traits as well. Although the great majority of schizoid persons commit no crimes and live either at the margins of society as night watchmen or in certain reclusive occupations, a few, by virtue of their extreme detachment from ordinary human feelings, become capable of crimes, including murder, that shock and horrify the public.

The most well-known example from contemporary American life concerns the "Unabomber," Theodore Kaczynski, the schizoid/paranoid former math professor and "antitechnology" fanatic, who mailed letter bombs to some two dozen persons who, for Kaczynski, symbolized the high-technology age. Three of the victims died. Kaczynski, who lived in a tiny hut in a remote part of Montana, was described as shy, withdrawn, and aloof. According to a former college roommate, Patrick McIntosh, he was ". . . one of the strangest people I met at Harvard. He was so intent on not being in contact with people even then" (Morganthau et al. 1996). The use of anonymous, mailed bombs is itself a clue to the likely schizoid nature of the perpetrator, because of the distance and lack of human contact between the bomber and his victims. A similar detachment is noted in a number of other "long-distance" poison-murders committed by schizoid psychopaths. Examples include Graham Young, who killed four persons in England with thallium poison (Holden 1995), and George Trepal, the schizoid and psychopathic chemist in Georgia who killed a neighbor woman, and almost killed her children, also using the tasteless, odorless thallium (Good and Goreck 1995), which he managed to secrete in the family's Coca-Cola bottles. Trepal had grown up as an aloof "computer nerd," having no friends of either sex; later on he was arrested for the manufacture of methamphetamines. He had built a secret torture chamber in the basement of his house, where he watched sadistic films about Ilse Koch (the commandant of Buchenwald concentration camp) and maintained his chemistry lab.

Paranoid traits were important elements in these schizoid murderers. Besides being aloof, for example, they were also mistrustful, secretive, grudge-bearing, and suspicious. There are abundant examples from the forensic literature, however, where paranoid personality disorder is the most prominent personality feature.

Paranoid Personality in Relation to Murder

Paranoid personality may operate down any one of several avenues as a predisposing factor to homicide. Many fanatics (including political terrorists) have an underlying paranoid personality structure, as was implicit in Kurt Schneider's appellation, "fanatic personality," for what we now call "paranoid." Schneider (1923/1950) mentioned *combative, aggressive,* and *litigious* as key traits. Murders committed by paranoid political and religious fanatics, including those who bomb abortion clinics or kill congregants at churches, temples, and mosques, are legion. Even the notably peaceful philosophy of Buddhism can get twisted into a lethal form, as was witnessed with Asahara and the followers of his Aum Shinri Kyoh movement in contemporary Japan.

Pathological jealousy, where one spouse is obsessed with, and mistakenly convinced of, the infidelity of the other spouse, is a common antecedent to murder. An example is that of Richard Minns, a wealthy health-spa tycoon (Finstad 1991) who abandoned his wife and four children to embark on an affair with Barbra Piotrowski, a beauty queen/premed student half his age. A ruthless businessman, Minns was described by those who knew him in these terms: paranoid, arrogant, egotistical, vengeful, violent, jealous, unethical, sensation-seeking, greedy, and mendacious. The affair took on the dimensions of a grand passion until Minns sabotaged the relationship through his virtual enslavement of Barbra, his lying (he didn't tell her he was married), and his stinginess (he wouldn't make a reasonable divorce settlement with his wife). Barbra eventually rebelled; Minns suspected she was "fooling around" with other men. After he punched her a few times, she packed and moved out. He then hired hit men to kill her. They succeeded only in rendering her paraplegic. Minns meantime escaped to Europe, where he has been in hiding ever since the attempted murder in 1982.

Pathological jealousy as a motive in the murder of women by estranged husbands or lovers—who violate orders of protection and then kill their quarry—is routine fare in the tabloids and affects persons in every walk of life. The famous *Tarasoff* case in California, which set the stage for the law that now requires mental health professionals to warn persons whom their patients speak of planning to harm or kill, revolved around the tenuous relationship between an immigrant, Prosenjit Poddar, and the young woman he admired from afar, and whom he mistakenly assumed was his "fiancée." She had handled (then tossed away) a gift he had left at her door, which in his culture signified engagement. Despondent and increasingly paranoid in the aftermath of this "rejection," he saw a psychiatrist and spoke of his urge to kill the Tarasoff girl, which he eventually did (Blum 1986).

Smoldering rage and resentment, coupled with a sense of "righteous indignation," combine to form another variety of paranoid personality. Men with this disposition, fired from their jobs for example, tend to feel unjustly picked on or mistreated and, in the extreme cases, make the headlines by gunning down the boss and all who happen to be in the way at the time, or else by killing as many innocents as possible in a restaurant or school or some other public place.

The case of the Chinese graduate student, Lu Gang (Lu being the family name), is an example (Chen 1995). Lu Gang was working on his Ph.D. in physics at the University of Iowa. Described as a "misfit" and morose loner, he alienated people, though he did brilliantly in his studies. But he was not as brilliant as another student from the Chinese mainland, who just edged out Lu for a certain physics prize. Lu became progressively paranoid about the professors in the physics department, believing that they were conspiring to humiliate him and deny him his merited award. At that juncture, Lu obtained a pistol permit and then calmly shot to death the physics chairman, his mentor, another professor, his countryman-rival, and a college dean whom he felt was "dismissive" of the paranoid screeds he wrote in efforts to have the prize switched to himself.

Prosenjit Poddar and Lu Gang both manifested paranoid, schizoid, and narcissistic traits, but without antisociality or psychopathy as commonly defined.

A somewhat more complex personality picture was that of the mass murderer Joseph Wesbecker, who killed eight co-workers at his printing plant when the foreman refused to place him in a less stressful work position. Wesbecker had engaged in some antisocial behaviors as an adolescent: arrests for disorderly conduct, siphoning gas from a truck, and intimidating girls with a starter-gun. But he worked very responsibly in the printing plant for many years, though becoming increasingly irritable over the pressures of the job. He also became "paranoid" about his wife's daughters by her first marriage, and then about his foreman, whom he saw as trying to drive him toward suicide by keeping him at his job as "folder" at a high-speed rotogravure press. Wesbecker was hospitalized several times for "manic depression" or "schizoaffective disorder" and eventually was given Prozac (fluoxetine) shortly before the massacre. Wesbecker was killed by the police during that encounter. The lawsuit mounted (unsuccessfully) by the survivors of the victims maintained that Prozac had "made him do it" (Cornwell 1996).

Borderline Personality and Its Relation to Murder

The descriptors of the DSM definition of BPD emphasize depression and irritability (lability of affect, recurrent suicidal behavior, inordinate anger, impulsivity). Violence directed against others is more common, as is self-directed violence, in those with BPD than in the general population. In my long-term follow-up study of 206 patients with BPD, 95% of whom were traced (the female-to-male ratio was 3:1), 4 had committed murder during the 10- to 25-year follow-up interval. All were males. One, who had been in a lifelong battle with parents who humiliated him constantly, killed his mother when he was 40, after she had refused him his favorite meal at Thanksgiving (Stone 1990). Another—an adolescent boy of 15—had burned down the house of a family whose son, the patient assumed, had molested his sister sexually. The other boy was on a sleep-away and was unharmed; his parents and brother died in the fire.

Females with BPD, though they outnumber their male counterparts considerably, and despite their tempestuousness, seldom commit murder, probably because women are much less likely to be antisocial or psychopathic than are men. The women diagnosed with BPD who do kill, do so often with the same flamboyance that characterizes every other aspect of their lives. A case in point: Laurie Wasserman Dann (Kaplan et al. 1990), who besides being diagnosed with BPD was also diagnosed with ASPD, obsessive-compulsive disorder, manic-depressive illness, and paranoid personality disorder, decompensated and went into a bizarre descent after her divorce from Russell Dann, whom she stabbed with an icepick while he slept. She had a consultation with a famous psychiatrist in the Chicago area, whose sensible recommendations she ignored. More than that, she sent him a container of fruit juice laced with poison, which he wisely declined to drink. In a final act of fury, she barged into the kindergarten of a Winnetka, Illinois, school, killing one child and wounding several others. As the police later closed in on her, she killed herself.

More than half the women with BPD whose murders have inspired full-length biographies (8 of 15 in my series) have been incest victims. This was the case with the North Carolinian farm girl Velma Barfield, the last woman to be legally executed in the United States. As she mentioned in her autobiography (Barfield 1985), her father had intercourse with her from when she was 13 until she married at 17. After her husband died a few years later from alcoholism, Velma became addicted to psychotropic drugs. At first she would falsify checks or steal small amounts to support her habit. Eventually she faked her mother's signature on a loan against her mother's house, and then poisoned her mother so she would never learn of the forgery. Unlike most of the other women with BPD who have murdered, Velma Barfield was not psychopathic, and not antisocial until she became addicted after the death of her husband.

Far more novelistic is the story of Darci Pierce (Hughes 1992), the Oregon adoptee who grew up hating her biological mother for giving her up and her adoptive mother for being obese and mean. Darci had rage outbursts at home from her earliest days, developed pseudologia fantastica, became cunningly manipulative, and carried on sexual relationships with several relatives from age 6 on. In adolescence she mutilated herself and made up stories of living in mansions and of taking fabulous trips. Her personality features, besides the borderline, were narcissistic/ grandiose, antisocial, and histrionic. Obsessed with the idea of having a baby and of proving herself a better mother than either of hers, she fooled her boyfriend, Ray Pierce, into marrying her because she was "pregnant." As the lie was about to get exposed (she even pretended to go to an obstetrician), she grew desperate and killed a nine months' pregnant woman, upon whom she did a cesarean section off a deserted highway, using a car key as scalpel, and then drove to a hospital, as though the hastily delivered baby were hers.

Sadistic Personality Disorder: A Still Useful Distinction

Sadistic personality disorder (SPD) has become a personality non grata in DSM. Relegated to the appendix of the 1980 and 1987 versions, it was abandoned altogether in DSM-IV. There had been eight descriptors originally; namely, 1) uses physical cruelty or violence to establish dominance, 2) humiliates or demeans people in the presence of others, 3) uses harsh discipline of a child or spouse, 4) takes pleasure in the suffering of others, 5) lies in order to inflict pain, 6) intimidates, 7) restricts others' autonomy, and 8) is fascinated by violence, weapons, torture, martial arts, or injury.

None of the SPD items overlaps with the defining features of ASPD, so it would not be legitimate to claim that the existence of ASPD in DSM-IV obviates the need for a separate SPD category. How SPD came to be eliminated from the manual (though not yet from human society) is an issue I will comment on later.

Persons with pronounced sadistic tendencies rarely seek psychotherapy, and thus lie largely outside the clinical experience of most psychiatrists, apart from those immersed in forensic work. This helps to account for the paucity of clinical trials and field work relevant to the disorder. The forensic psychologist Reid Meloy has made several contributions to the topic (S. E. Holt, J. R. Meloy, and S. Strack, unpublished manuscript, 1996; Meloy 1992, unpublished manuscript, 1996). In a study of 41 inmates at a maximum security prison, Holt et al. divided the participants into a group with psychopathy (by the PCL-R) and a nonpsychopathic group. Sadistic tendencies were assessed using the Millon Clinical Multiaxial Inventory-II, Scale 6-B (1987). Psychopaths were found to be significantly more sadistic than nonpsychopaths. Sadism, in Holt et al.'s study, did not differentiate the violent men (whose acts did not involve sex) from the sexually violent men. It should be noted that the PCL-R items also do not overlap with the DSM-III/III-R definition of SPD, although both DSM-IV and PCL-R include the trait: "lack of remorse." Lack of remorse, by itself, does not differentiate sadistic from nonsadistic persons, inasmuch as one can readily envision an embezzler or a jewel thief who lacks remorse. Although childhood physical or sexual abuse is common in the histories of psychopaths and of serial sexual killers (Ressler et al. 1988; Stone 1994), many of the 34 criminal sexual sadists studied by Dietz et al. (1990) had not experienced abuse during childhood. It is the emphasis on the exaction and subsequent enjoyment of another's suffering that distinguishes SPD from other aberrations of personality, especially when we recognize that only a proportion of psychopaths are in addition *sadistic*. Actually, a sexual sadistic murderer whom Dietz had interviewed supplied Dietz with an even more compelling definition of sadism, coming as it did from the offender himself: "The wish to inflict pain is not the essence of sadism. One essential impulse: To have complete mastery over another person. . . . The most radical aim is to make her suffer since there is no greater power over another person than that of inflicting pain . . ." (p. 165). Of the 30 sexually sadistic criminals Dietz and his colleagues studied intensively, 28 had carefully planned their offenses, and 27 used a "con" approach to lure their victims. All of these men could be diagnosed, in effect, as narcissistic and sadistic psychopaths. The authors point out that there are ". . . far larger numbers of sexual sadists who commit less extreme crimes" (p. 173). The extreme cases— the serial sexual killers—differ from the less destructive sexual sadists ". . . not in the severity of the paraphilia, but in the character pathology that permits them such uninhibited expression of their sexual desires" (p. 173). This led Dietz to speculate that NPD and psychopathy were on a continuum, with psychopathy representing an extreme example of narcissistic pathology. As is clear from remarks earlier in this chapter, I am wholeheartedly in accord with this view.

My own information and impressions regarding sadistic personality derive mainly from two sources: my work at a forensic psychiatric hospital, and my analysis of some 297 (as of this writing) full-length biographies of murderers, some of which have been reported on elsewhere (Stone 1993). Using the DSM-III criteria, I could establish that 196 of the 299 murderers fulfilled the minimum of four, or more, of SPD criteria: 173 of the 243 males (71%), and 23 of the 56 females (41%) ($\chi^2 = 18.3$, $P < .001$). It is to be expected that SPD would be more common in males, and this is even more true if we focus on the group of serial killers. This expectation relates to the greater propensity of males to behave aggressively, based on the differential effects of testosterone levels in the two sexes (Valzelli 1981). This difference apparently also contributes to the much higher likelihood of ASPD to be diagnosed in males than in females (Robins et al. 1984).

In my series of serial killers, 71 of the 77 males met criteria for SPD. Almost all (74 of the 77) met PCL-R criteria for psychopathy, using scores of 25 or higher. Sexual sadism (DSM-IV: 302.84) was a feature of all the male serial killers, with the exception of four (including the notorious "Son of Sam": David Berkowitz

[Klausner 1981]), and was not a feature of the three female serial killers. Among the males, 37 of the serial killers were schizoid (48%), making the constellation *sadistic, psychopathic,* and *schizoid* a particularly common personality profile in serial sexual homicide. The seemingly high proportion of male serial sexual killers who are also psychopaths (74/77 or 96%) is, incidentally, in line with the observations of Yarvis (1995), who studied a group of 180 men who were either murderers, rapists, or "rapist/ murderers" (30% of whom also carried the diagnosis of sexual sadism). ASPD was noted in a quarter of the murderers and 18% of the rapists, but in 90% of the rapist/murderers. In Yarvis's survey the next most common personality disorder was BPD, found in a fifth of the murderers and in a third of the rapists, but in none of the rapist/murderers (p. 414). This finding also mirrors my own impressions: Of the 77 biographied serial killers in my series, only John Wayne Gacy (Cahill 1986) was diagnosed "borderline" (by a court-appointed psychiatrist) in 1979, before the appearance of DSM-III. "Borderline" was used at that time as roughly equivalent to *pseudoneurotic schizophrenia* (the diagnosis preferred by the defense psychiatrist). But even Gacy would not meet DSM-III or DSM-IV criteria for BPD, though he would for either ASPD or psychopathy.

The distribution of personality disorders in a forensic psychiatric hospital apparently differs from that of the biographied murderer series. I have thus far examined 30 men remanded to a forensic unit at the Mid-Hudson Psychiatric Center. Of these, 17 were admitted because of a previous murder (10), attempted murder (6), or vehicular homicide (1). Only 6 met PCL-R criteria for psychopathy (with scores of 25 or greater), including the 3 serial/sexual murderers. Ten met DSM-IV criteria for ASPD, and 10 met criteria for paranoid PD. Three were schizoid (the serial killers were not schizoid), and none showed BPD. Many of the men had been called "schizophrenic" before coming to Mid-Hudson, but abuse of psychotomimetic drugs was at the root of most of this faux-schizophrenia. There were only 2 with unequivocal schizophrenia, 1 with manic-depression, and 1 with a depressive psychosis.

Comments and Discussion

The preceding remarks and data derive from the biographical material mentioned earlier, from my experience on a forensic psychiatric unit, and from review of the literature. The literature reflects for the most part studies carried out either in prisons or in forensic hospitals, or in the courtroom. The recent literature has often been embellished by access to modern computerized data on violent crime accumulated for the Federal Bureau of Investigation. Even pooled, this literature can only be said to open a few windows onto the personality profiles of those who murder. Magazine articles and newspaper clippings of murders, both the notorious and the mundane, constitute another source, although in the several hundred such in my own files, only a few are detailed enough to shed light on the subtleties of personality. In a country where more than 20,000 murders occur annually, many make the local papers, but, as mentioned, only the more dramatic inspire lengthy treatises of the sort that allow distinctions about personality subtypes to be made. Suffice it to say that a personality disorder of some type is present in the great majority of persons who murder. The largest fraction of murders stems from impulsive, spur-of-the-moment aggressive acts; the personality disorders that underlie such acts are likely to be irritable/explosive, paranoid, and occasionally borderline or depressive. In a famous case of *crime passionel*, Jean Harris (1986), when betrayed by her lover, the "Scarsdale Diet" doctor, Abe Tarnower, became severely depressed and enraged, in which state she shot the "two-timing" doctor to death. She had led an exemplary life up until then and was certainly not psychopathic. Most *crimes passionels* are committed by nonpsychopathic persons, who are much less likely to kill again upon release from incarceration than are murderers whose PCL scores are in the highest decile (Sreenivasan et al. 1997; Villeneuve and Quinsey 1995).

The many murders committed by impulse-ridden or grudge-holding persons seldom see more than a few days reportage in the local newspapers. These usually involve persons with explosive or paranoid traits. Mass murderers may have either or both of these qualities. Richard Speck (Altman and Ziporyn 1967), who stabbed eight nurses to death (while a ninth, hiding under a bed, looked on), was psychopathic and explosive/irritable. Michael Ryan, who shot to death 16 people (including his mother) in Hungerford, England, was a schizoid "misfit," an abrasive and increasingly paranoid loner who made up fanciful stories about sexual conquests he never made, until he "blew" in August of 1987, shooting at random with his AK-47 (Josephs 1993). Less is actually known about the intimate details of mass murderers' personalities, since, as with Ryan, Charles Whitman of the Texas Tower massacre, and others, most are killed either by the police or by themselves and do not face extensive scrutiny at trial.

Spousal murders, or more generally, murder of intimate sexual partners, fall into two broad classes: those fueled by jealousy (whether justified or delusional) in persons of a paranoid personality bent, or else those prompted by the desire to rid oneself of a "burdensome" spouse in order to be with a new lover. Here the personality is often psychopathic, or at least strong psychopathic trends can be discerned. The case of the debt-ridden, Tom's River, New Jersey, husband Rob Marshall is illustrative: He fell in love with a wealthy neighbor, took out a large life-insurance policy on his wife (with himself as the beneficiary), and then hired a hit man to kill her. Marshall had many psychopathic traits, as McGinnis (1989) makes clear in his biography.

Hare (1996) has demonstrated good correlations between elevated PCL scores and failure to remain out of prison after release: In one 3-year follow-up study, 75% of nonpsychopaths had not been reincarcerated, whereas only 20% of the psychopaths remained out of prison (p. 40). Psychopathic murderers are particularly prone to kill again if their initial victim(s) were strangers, as is the case routinely in serial sexual homicide.

Serial killers, especially the large subgroup who are motivated by sexual sadism, show psychopathic and sadistic personalities; some of the more grotesque murders by such persons are committed by those with concomitant schizoid personality (Jeffrey Dahmer was an example [Schwartz 1992]).

The presence of marked sadistic traits renders the prognosis for social recovery even less likely than is the case for nonsadistic but psychopathic murderers, in whom the recovery rate is already vanishingly small. Many of the serious mistakes made in the premature release (or release at all) of men who go on to commit further murders stem from the failure to take into account clear-cut evidence of prior sadistic behavior. Gary Taylor (Imbrie 1993) is a case in point. Taylor, who grew up in Detroit, used to assault women from the time he was 13 on, also hurling objects at them or shooting them with a BB gun. Later he impersonated an FBI agent and raped several women. Incarcerated finally, he was put through an alcohol-treatment program, and, though diagnosed "sociopathic," he was released from Ypsilanti Forensic Hospital, so long as he promised to check in with the hospital periodically. Taylor instead returned to his old ways, only with a vengeance, becoming a serial sexual killer, who buried his victims in a specially built torture chamber in his house.

Although it is most rare for sexual sadists who become serial killers to be psychotic—only 2 in my series of 77 were (Philadelphia's Joseph Kallinger [Schreiber 1984] and Ed Gein [Gollmar 1981])—the horrendous nature of their crimes ensures that they are sent to a conventional prison rather than to a forensic psychiatric hospital. The latter is viewed by the public as too "soft" a berth for killers of that stripe. And in general, prisons contain a higher proportion of offenders with pronounced psychopathic personalities than would be found in a forensic hospital. Likewise, the proportion of markedly sadistic offenders is greater in the prison setting.

Given the conceptual distinction between psychopathy and sadistic personality, and in view of the significance of sadism in relation to the serious risks of either violent assault or murder, how, we may ask, do we justify the exclusion of SPD from our standard nomenclature? Answers to this question have been put forward by Thomas Widiger and by Robert Spitzer. Widiger (1996) mentioned the concern that consultants helping to revise DSM felt concerning the use zealous defense attorneys might make of SPD, were it placed within the DSM. Violent sadistic felons might be released or given light sentences on the grounds of "diminished capacity" or "mental illness," if their attorneys construed SPD as an "illness" exculpating their clients of the crimes committed. To squelch such opportunism in the courtroom, SPD was dropped from the manual. Widiger alluded to the paradoxical situation in which feminist consultants who were the most forceful in condemning the sadistic practices by which certain men subjugated women were also the most alarmed by the possibility that the diagnosis could be misused to exculpate such men (or, at least, lighten their sentences). Spitzer et al. (1991) carried out a survey of psychiatrists on this thorny topic and found that three-quarters of the respondents worried about a similar misuse of SPD in forensic settings—leading to the "medicalization of evil deeds." The respondents feared that inclusion of this personality diagnosis would trivialize its impact, sanitizing sadistic acts as though they were merely the by-product of an "illness." I can envision a more sensible approach to this admittedly touchy social and political issue. Has the time not come for the psychiatric profession to make it abundantly clear to the legal community that sadistic personalities, while lamentably they surely exist, are for all intents and purposes untreatable (especially when the person in question has already embarked upon a career of sadistically violating other people) and not to be viewed as an illness justifying exculpation or reduction of sentence? Were psychiatry to take a firm stand regarding this most ominous of all the personality configurations, our taxonomy would be more true to what exists in nature, and our position would be more enlightened within the forensic domain.

References

Altman KR, Ziporyn M: Born to Raise Hell: The Untold Story of Richard Speck. New York, Grove Press, 1967

American Psychiatric Association: Diagnostic and Statistical Manual of Mental Disorders, 3rd Edition. Washington, DC, American Psychiatric Association, 1980

American Psychiatric Association: Diagnostic and Statistical Manual of Mental Disorders, 3rd Edition, Revised. Washington, DC, American Psychiatric Association, 1987

American Psychiatric Association: Diagnostic and Statistical Manual of Mental Disorders, 4th Edition. Washington, DC, American Psychiatric Association, 1994

Andersen HS, Sestoft D, Lillebaek T, et al: Prevalence of ICD-10 psychiatric morbidity in samples of prisoners on remand. Int J Law Psychiatry 19:61–74, 1996

Barfield V: Woman on Death Row. Minneapolis, World Wide Publications, 1985

Blum D: Bad Karma: A True Story of Obsession and Murder. New York, Atheneum, 1986

Cahill T: Buried Dreams: Inside the Mind of a Serial Killer. New York, Bantam Books, 1986

Chen E: Deadly Scholarship: The True Story of Lu Gang and Mass Murder in America's Heartland. New York, Birch Lane Press, 1995

Cleckley H: The Mask of Sanity, 5th Edition. St. Louis, CV Mosby, 1972

Cornwell J: The Power to Harm: Mind, Medicine and Murder on Trial. New York, Viking Press, 1996

Dietz PE, Hazelwood R, Warren J: The sexually sadistic criminal and his offenses. Bull Am Acad Psychiatry Law 18:163–178, 1990

Dunne D: Courtroom notebook: the Menendez murder trial. Vanity Fair, October 1993, pp 252ff

Eronen M, Hakola P, Tiihonen J: Mental disorders and homicidal behavior in Finland. Arch Gen Psychiatry 53:497–501, 1996

Finstad S: Sleeping With the Devil. New York, Wm. Morrow, 1991

Geberth VJ, Turco RN: Antisocial personality disorder, sexual sadism, malignant narcissism, and serial murder. J Forensic Sc 42:49–60, 1997

Gollmar RH: Ed Gein: America's Most Bizarre Murderer. New York, Windsor Publishing, 1981

Good J, Goreck S: Poison Mind: The True Story of the Mensa Murderer—and the Policewoman Who Risked Her Life to Bring Him to Justice. New York, Wm. Morrow, 1995

Hare RD: Psychopathy: a construct whose time has come. Crim Justice Behav 23:25–54, 1996

Hare RD, Harpur TJ, Hakstian AR, et al: The revised Psychopathy Checklist: reliability and factor structure. Psychological Assessment 2:338–341, 1990

Harpur TJ, Hakstian R, Hare RD: Factor structure of the Psychopathy Checklist. J Consult Clin Psychol 56:741–747, 1988

Harris J: Stranger in Two Worlds. New York, Zebra Press, 1986

Holden A: The Saint Albans Poisoner. London, Corgi Books, 1995

Hughes DT: Lullaby and Good Night. New York, Pocket Books, 1992

Imbrie AE: Spoken in Darkness. New York, Plume Books, 1993

Josephs J: Hungerford: One Man's Massacre. London, Smith-Gryphon, 1993

Kaplan J, Papajohn G, Zorn E: Murder of Innocence: The Tragic Life & Final Rampage of Laurie Dann. New York, Warner Books, 1990

Klausner LD: Son of Sam. New York, McGraw-Hill, 1981

Kraepelin E: Psychiatrie, 8th Edition, Vol 4. Leipzig, J. A. Barth Verlag, pp 1909–1915

Maclean H: In Broad Daylight: A Murder in Skidmore, Missouri. New York, Harper & Row, 1988

McGinnis J: Blind Faith. New York, Putnam, 1989

Meloy JR: Violent Attachments. Northvale, NJ, Aronson, 1992

Millon T: Millon Clinical Multiaxial Inventory-II Manual. Minneapolis, National Computer Systems, 1987

Morganthau T, Hosenball M, Miller M, et al: Probing the mind of a killer. Newsweek, April 15, 1996

Oldham JM, Skodol AE, Kellman HD, et al: Diagnosis of DSM-III-R personality disorder by two structured interviews: patterns of co-morbidity. Am J Psychiatry 149:213–220, 1992

Rasmussen K, Levander S: Symptoms and personality characteristics of patients in a maximum security unit. Int J Law Psychiatry 18:117–127, 1995

Ressler RK, Burgess AW, Douglas JE: Sexual Homicide: Patterns & Motives. New York, Macmillan, 1988

Rice ME, Harris GT: Psychopathy, schizophrenia, alcohol abuse and violent recidivism. Int J Law Psychiatry 18:333–342, 1995

Robins LN, Helzer JE, Weissman MM, et al: Lifetime prevalence of specific psychiatric disorders in three sites. Arch Gen Psychiatry 41:949–958, 1984

Schneider K: Psychopathic Personalities. London, Cassell, 1923/1950

Schreiber FR: The Shoemaker: The Anatomy of a Psychotic. New York, Signet Books, 1984

Schwartz A: The Man Who Could Not Kill Enough: The Secret Murders of Milwaukee's Jeffrey Dahmer. New York, Carol Publishing, 1992

Serin RC, Amos NL: The role of psychopathy in the assessment of dangerousness. Int J Law Psychiatry 18:231–238, 1995

Smith C: Seeds of Evil—A True Story of Murder and Money in California. New York, St. Martin's, 1997

Spitzer L, Fiester SJ, Gay M, et al: Is sadistic personality disorder a valid diagnosis? Am J Psychiatry 148:875–879, 1991

Sreenivasan S, Kirkish P, Eth S, et al: Predictors of recidivistic violence in criminally insane and civilly committed psychiatric inpatients. Int J Law Psychiatry 20:279–291, 1997

Stone MH: The Fate of Borderlines. New York, Guilford Press, 1990

Stone MH: Abnormalities of Personality: Within & Beyond the Realm of Treatment. New York, WW Norton, 1993

Stone MH: Early traumatic factors in the lives of serial murderers. Am J Forensic Psychiatry 15:5–26, 1994

Valzelli L: Psychobiology of Aggression and Violence. New York, Raven, 1981

Villeneuve DB, Quinsey VL: Predictors of general and violent recidivism among mentally disordered inmates. Crim Justice Behav 22:397–410, 1995

Widiger TA: Aggression: within and beyond the DSM-IV. Presented at the 149th annual meeting of the American Psychiatric Association, New York, May 9, 1996

Wolfgang ME: Homicide in other industrialized countries. Bull N Y Acad Sci 62:400–412, 1986

Yarvis RM: Diagnostic patterns among three violent offender types. Bull Am Acad Psychiatry Law 23:411–419, 1995

Chapter 3

Axis II Disorders and Motivation for Serious Criminal Behavior

Jeremy W. Coid, M.D., F.R.C.Psych.

The relationship between the Axis II personality disorders and serious criminal behavior has been a relatively neglected area of research. Individuals with personality disorder are traditionally considered to constitute a significant proportion of the mentally disordered violent (Krakowski et al. 1986). However, many health care professionals continue to debate whether psychiatric treatment is an appropriate use of limited resources following serious offenses by individuals with severe personality disorder, especially as the evidence for the effectiveness of current therapies remains equivocal for those with psychopathic and antisocial traits (Dolan and Coid 1993). Nevertheless, the mental health legislation of many countries does permit the treatment of offenders with mental disorders in a hospital setting as an alternative to imprisonment or following transfer to hospital during a prison sentence. For example, less than 1% of all compulsory admissions to general psychiatric hospitals in England and Wales receive a primary diagnosis of personality disorder, but in the maximum- and medium-secure forensic psychiatry services, 16% receive this diagnosis. An understanding of the offending behavior of these patients and its relationship to Axis II psychopathology is therefore essential in their assessment, selection for treatment, and subsequent management.

Future research in this area has major implications for developments in four main areas. First, research may have influence in the refinement of forensic assessments of offender patients and where mental health care professionals have a major role in providing advice to courts when determining an offender's responsibility for a criminal act. Second, understanding the motivation for offending behavior may have a crucial bearing on the choice of treatment that should be offered to these patients, the level of security required in which to deliver treatment, and in some cases may be relevant to the likelihood of a successful response to the treatment. Third, associations between criminal behavior and personality psychopathology may be highly important in the assessment of risk of future reoffending. And, finally, research in this area may ultimately contribute to more effective criminal profiling and behavioral assessments being carried out during criminal investigations.

Assessment of Offenders and Criminal Behavior

There are few established and tested theoretical models that can guide research into the relationship between personality disorder and the dynamics of serious criminal behavior. In clinical practice, mental health evaluations of offenders typically involve the deconstruction of the criminal act, examining the various identified components in relation to identified psychopathology. But when attempting to empirically test the relationship between the two, there are a series of problems. Criminal behavior is defined by law. Within most jurisdictions, motivation does not necessarily affect legal liability or the ultimate finding of guilt (although motive is always relevant in evidence and may be highly important in the consideration of appropriate punishment). Thus, legal theory, although it defines the act, may have little to offer in the empirical study of the associations between personality and crime. Criminal behavior is also highly complex. This poses a major challenge when creating variables that can measure the various components of the criminal act for subsequent examination in relation to Axis II psychopathology. For example, criminal behavior could be broken down into characteristics that describe the act itself, characteristics of the offender and victim, motives or motivating factors that induced the offender to act in a certain way, and additional shaping factors, such as disinhibiting influences of intoxication, incitement or encouragement from others, and so on. A dynamic relationship can clearly exist among several of these factors within a single act. Furthermore, the time frame for each of these interactions, and the addition of external circumstances, may cause further difficulties. Finally, some offending behaviors and Axis II psychopathology have a direct link; for example, repetitive impulsive behaviors, the orchestration of circumstances that lead to interpersonal conflicts, and the tendency to experience intense affects or paranoid ideation when under stress.

This chapter presents a brief overview of the main themes within previous research into the associations between criminal behavior, motivation, and abnormalities of personality. However, it will become apparent that there has been little research into the associations with abnormality of personality as defined within the DSM Axis II disorders. The chapter therefore presents new data that examine the independent associations between DSM-III Axis II disorders, lifetime Axis I disorders, and a second set of motivating and shaping influences observed within the dynamics of serious crimes of violence, sexual offenses, and arson in a sample of convicted prisoners and patients detained in maximum security hospitals in England. To test these associations, it has been necessary to devise a taxonomy of motivating factors for the study; these are described in an appendix to this chapter.

Personality Disorder and Criminal Behavior

Violent Crime

The situational approach to understanding violent criminal behavior is established in the psychological literature as one that seeks to analyze the environmental factors associated with violent acts (Monahan and Klassen 1982). Hollin (1989) has reviewed the studies that have focused on the context in which crimes of serious assault, robbery, and murder occur. Several researchers have attempted to create a typology of violent incidents using factors such as the type of violence used, characteristics of the victim, location of the assault, and so on. These variables have also been used to classify types of violent offender, sometimes incorporating the intention of the individual when carrying out the offense. Although this approach can be helpful in demonstrating that different people commit violent crimes for different reasons and under different conditions, it does not say much about the person involved. Hollin concludes that a more detailed assessment of the behavior, in conjunction with specific characteristics of the offender, is ultimately required.

A body of literature has attempted to investigate the psychology of the violent offender by examining the links between personality and violence. An early model was proposed by Megargee (1966) in which violence was hypothesized to occur when the instigation to violence, mediated by anger, would exceed the individual's level of control of aggressive feelings or impulses. An "undercontrolled" person would have very low inhibitors and would therefore frequently act in a violent manner if provocation was perceived. On the other hand, an "overcontrolled" person would have extremely strong inhibitors, and violence would occur if the provocation had been intense or endured over a long period of time. Megargee predicted that an overcontrolled personality would be found in those who had committed acts of extreme violence, but not in those with histories of frequent minor assaults. Blackburn (1968) confirmed these predictions in a group of violent offenders, although Crawford (1977) failed to replicate the findings. Nevertheless, subsequent work by Quinsey et al. (1983) and Henderson (1983) has confirmed that there are deficiencies in the assertive behavior of overcontrolled offenders and that individuals with low psychometric measures of control report difficulty in controlling their temper and in avoiding fights.

Although the evidence appears to support the overcontrolled-undercontrolled dichotomy, more significant advances in the classification of offenders came in a series of later studies that searched for types, or clusters, based on scores of personality measures. Studies by Blackburn (1971, 1975, 1986) revealed four types of serious offender, including primary psychopaths, secondary psychopaths, controlled (nonpsychopathic) offenders, and inhibited (nonpsychopathic) offenders. These findings were

Does disorder = crime

replicated by McGurk (1978) and Henderson (1982). Neverthe-less, detailed information on the patterns and motivations of the offending behavior in relation to these personality types was lim-ited in these studies. However, there was some evidence that the inhibited and controlled groups had less history of repeated vi-olence than the two psychopathic groups, especially the primary psychopaths, consistent with the overcontrol hypothesis.

Blackburn (1989) argued that it is important to distinguish be-tween the occurrence of a violent act and a tendency to repeat such acts, because the act of violence in itself does not necessarily imply an aggressive personality. A trait of aggressiveness will imply consistency over time and place (Litwack and Schlesinger 1987). Aggressive personality traits are evident within the DSM Axis II typology. Traits essential to current clinical concepts of personality disorder are defined in DSM-IV as enduring patterns of perceiving, relating to, and thinking about the environment and oneself that are exhibited in a wide range of social and per-sonal contexts. When personality traits are inflexible and mala-daptive, they can cause significant functional impairment or sub-jective distress. Widiger and Trull (1994) pointed out that violent behavior is a defining feature of two of the personality disorders (borderline and antisocial), and antagonistic, hostile traits are evident in eight of the personality disorders (paranoid, anti-social, borderline, histrionic, narcissistic, passive-aggressive, schizotypal, and obsessive compulsive). Axis II disorders would appear to have considerable potential for contributing to the dy-namics of violent crime. But little evidence exists to confirm this possibility or to indicate the extent to which these individual diagnostic categories influence actions, motivations, choice of victim, or associated features of the criminal act.

In their review of the associations between personality disor-der and violence, Widiger and Trull (1994) confirmed a shortage of information in this area. They observed that antisocial per-sonality disorder and psychopathy increased the risk that an in-dividual will engage in violent behavior. However, this does not imply that the behavior can be predicted in any given time pe-riod. The review was highly critical of the DSM categorical ap-proach, arguing that quantitative scores of personality dimensions have superior psychometric properties, and promoted the five-factor model of personality (Digman 1990) as an alternative. Nevertheless, until there is empirical evidence of the superiority of dimensional measures, it may be premature to abandon the DSM Axis II categorization when assessing violent offenders.

Sexual Offending

Situational approaches to sexual offending have led to a series of descriptive analyses of offense characteristics (see review by Hollin 1989). In the case of rape, a range of strategies have been used in categorization, including specific aspects of the offense, characteristics of the victim, and psychiatric and legal subgroupings (Amir 1971; Gebhard et al. 1965; Gibbens et al. 1977; Henne et al. 1976; Rada 1978). An alternative approach is to classify the act according to the motives of the rapists (Box 1983; Cohen 1971; Groth 1979; Guttmacher 1951; Prentsky et al. 1985). However, none of these studies have examined the relationship between their classification and personality disorder, although it is readily apparent that several of these taxonomies could be usefully examined in relation to the Axis II classification. For example, Groth (1979) described three types of rape, according to varying degrees of hostility and control associated with the rape, that could be associated with individual personality traits or Axis II categories observed in the offender. "Anger" rape typically follows arguments, sexual jealousies, and social rejection. The offender typically reports experiencing anger and rage, together with feelings of being wrongly treated prior to the act. During the assault, the rapist uses more force than is necessary to inflict physical injury and with the rape as an additional way of inflicting pain. "Power" rape differs in that sexual conquest is the goal and where physical aggression is used as necessary to force compliance. In "sadistic" rape, sexuality and aggression are combined. The victim is often bound and helpless, is humiliated, and may be tortured, which also provides a source of sexual excitement for the rapist.

Prentsky et al. (1985) have described a more elaborate classification including eight types of rapist, according to combinations of the meaning of aggression for the offender, the meaning of sexuality, and the offender's level of impulsivity. Aggression during the act can be instrumental to enforce compliance or expressive, in which the act is primarily aggressive. The meaning of the sexuality in the act can be compensatory, where the behavior is used to act out a sexual fantasy; exploitative, in which the rape is a predatory act; displaced anger, in which it is an expression of rage; and sadistic, where it is the acting out of sadistic fantasies. Whether the meaning of the sexuality and aggression in the act is determined by Axis II psychopathology in the offender could be explored in further studies using this classification.

Ressler et al. (1988) have proposed a motivational model to explain sexual homicide. This comprises a more complex and detailed framework than used by previous authors and may hold considerable promise for future research. It also demonstrates parallels with the biosocial interaction hypothesis (Raine et al. 1994) of abnormal personality development. The model incorporates interacting components, including the murderer's social environment, child and adolescent formative events, patterned responses to these events, resulting actions toward others, and the killer's reactions via a mental "feedback" filter to his murderous acts. Within their model, Ressler and colleagues propose a series of processes that are closely interwoven with the offender's personality, which develop over the life span, leading up to the homicide, and with the origins of several components within the childhood environment. In some cases it is probable that constitutional abnormalities, including neurodevelopmental abnormality and genetic factors, make substantial contributions to the development of the offending behavior by interacting with environmental factors over the life span. Although this model is not a classification of sexual homicide, it provides a very useful description of the personality development of the offender and the closely interwoven quality of the motivating and shaping factors leading up to the homicidal behavior.

Constructing a Typology of Motivation

In the absence of a previously tested model to examine the relationship between Axis II disorders and the dynamics of criminal behavior, a descriptive model was developed specifically for this study. This was derived largely from clinical experience in the forensic assessment of offender patients. Improvements in the clinical assessment of individuals with severe personality disorder have previously been recommended using a "two-dimensional" approach in which personality disorder, clinical syndromes, and associated behavioral disorder are carried out simultaneously, but taking an additional lifetime perspective of these overlapping areas of psychopathology (Coid 1993a; Dolan and Coid 1993). For the purpose of simplification, the time frame for the offending behavior in this study had to be narrowed. The motivational factors that were described by the participants as operating immediately before, and the situational factors during, the commission of the criminal act were therefore recorded and subsequently examined in relation to the subject's psychopathology, the latter measured using Axis II and lifetime Axis I (clinical syndrome) categories. It was necessary to construct a new typology based on a range of motivational variables that had led to the behavior, the key situational variables, and to establish these and the relevant antecedents with the subject at interview. Certain categories were derived from previous research; for example, the motivational typology of rape as described in the last section. Although the new typology was intended to concentrate primarily on motivational variables, it was also necessary to include certain shaping factors, such as intoxication with drugs and/or alcohol, whether the offense was carried out in a gang or as a group activity, and so on. The definitions of each of the variables included in this taxonomy are included in this chapter's appendix.

Participants and Methods

The study participants consisted of 260 males and females detained in maximum security hospitals and prisons in England following serious offending. The collection of participants has been described in detail in a previous publication (Coid 1992). The location and specification of participants is shown in Table 3–1. In this table, "psychopaths" refers to the English Mental Health Act, 1983, legal category of psychopathic disorder that is broadly defined as "a persistent disorder of disability of mind (whether or not including significant impairment of intelligence) which results in abnormally aggressive or seriously irresponsible misconduct on the part of the person concerned." This should not be confused with Hare's (1991) construct of psychopathy measured using the Psychopathy Checklist. In the table, "deteriorated" refers to serious mental disorder. Several individuals had developed symptoms of chronic process schizophrenia following their admission or imprisonment, and a smaller number had developed organic conditions, although the original clinical assessment had made a primary diagnosis of personality disorder. Of the original target sample of 315 individuals, 25 (8%) refused to take part, 24 (8%) were interviewed but were unable to complete all questionnaires due to the presence of Axis I symptoms, and 6 (2%) were released or died before they could be interviewed.

All individuals were interviewed with the Structured Clinical

Table 3–1. Location and specification of subsamples

	Female psychopaths	Male psychopaths	Male prisoners
Location	Broadmoor, Rampton, Ashworth hospitals	Broadmoor Hospital	Parkhurst, Lincoln, Hull prisons
Specification	3 maximum security hospitals	1 maximum security hospital	3 special units for dangerous prisoners
Study period	1984–1987	1984–1986	1987–1993
Total sample	104	111	100
No. released/died	0	3 (3)	3 (3)
No. incomplete	10 (10)	8 (7)	6 (6)
No. interviewed	93 (89)	86 (78)	81 (81)

Note. Total sample size $N = 260$.

Interview for DSM-III Axis II disorders, first edition (SCID) (Spitzer and Williams 1983). Male participants were administered the Schedule for Affective Disorders and Schizophrenia–Lifetime Version (SADS-L) (Spitzer and Endicott 1978) and females the Diagnostic Interview Schedule (DIS) (Robins et al. 1981) to obtain lifetime DSM-III Axis I disorder. As the SADS-L provided research diagnostic criteria diagnoses, the data were reviewed and the diagnoses subsequently revised to DSM-III categories. Hesselbrock et al. (1982) have demonstrated a high degree of diagnostic concordance for most diagnostic categories between these two interview schedules. For the purpose of this study, minor depressive disorder in the SADS-L was excluded, because the threshold was considered too low for equivalent comparison with DSM-III depressive disorder. Schizoaffective disorder was not included in the DSM-III classification and schizophreniform disorder was not included in the Research Diagnostic Criteria (RDC) (Spitzer et al. 1978). Both were included under the category "schizophrenia" in this study. Unspecified psychosis did not appear in the DSM-III classification but appears in RDC as unspecified functional psychosis. During the process of data collection, the DSM-III was revised to DSM-III-R and the SCID underwent further refinement by Spitzer and colleagues. However, the original instruments were retained for diagnostic continuity within the study.

Each subject was interviewed for a minimum of 3.5 hours by the author. Nurses or prison staff were also interviewed to obtain their opinion and to clarify data on each subject. In most cases, witness statements were available describing the offending behavior, and this was discussed in detail with the subject. All participants who had previously been in a psychiatric hospital or who had attended outpatients had their case notes requested for further examination. Reports were also requested from special schools, other institutions in which they had been resident in the past, and the probation service when relevant.

It was important to be fully aware of the details of the index offense leading to imprisonment or hospital admission before interviewing the participant. The majority of individuals were entirely frank about the facts of their crime, but a subgroup of the participants were evasive or would minimize the seriousness of their crime. In several individuals, relevant antecedents, such as sadistic masturbatory fantasies, compulsive homicidal urges, and pyromania, emerged for the first time. The interview established the situational context of the offense and the actions of the offender and victim, together with the offender's feelings at the time and intentions, based on his or her retrospective account. The interview essentially involved the construction of a narrative in which the offender relived the offense.

Statistical Analysis

To minimize confounding between diagnostic categories, both within and between the axes, the data analysis involved two separate stages: first, computation of the odds ratios of association and, second, the adjustment of these odds ratios using logistic regression. The first stage involved cross-tabulations in the form of intercorrelation matrices between different sets of values. These included cross-tabulations for Axis I–Axis I, Axis II–Axis II, and Axis II–Axis I as well as cross-tabulations between the motivational variables. To establish the statistical associations between these categorical variables, both χ^2 and odds ratios were used within the comparison tables. However, certain statistical associations between these variables in this first stage could have been spurious due to confounding. The second stage of the analysis therefore employed logistic regression, using a forward stepwise method (Wald) using SPSS.

Covariates were systematically entered into a stepwise procedure. These were obtained from the first stage of data analysis and the first intercorrelation matrix that showed odds ratios and χ^2 levels of significance. The mutually co-occurring factors derived from this first analysis were then entered into the second stage, logistic regression. Covariates were entered when the odds ratio of their association equaled 2.0 or more, .5 or less, or when the level of the χ^2 significance equaled more than .05. Following logistic regression, a final intercorrelation matrix was constructed, consisting of the adjusted odds ratios, now controlled for confounders from both diagnostic axes. When there were no mutually co-occurring potential confounders, the original odds ratio from the first phase of analysis was entered into this final matrix. The tables shown in this chapter are a summary of the main findings of interest that were derived from the second-phase matrix tables.

Results

DSM-III Axis II Personality Disorders

Borderline personality disorder was the most common Axis II disorder in the overall sample, followed by antisocial disorder in just half the participants (see Table 3–2). However, most individuals received multiple Axis II categories with an overall mean of 3.6 (SD, 1.8; range, 0–9). Categories such as passive-aggressive, avoidant, compulsive, and self-defeating personality disorder were never found as a single diagnosis. The small subgroup without any Axis II diagnosis was highly heterogeneous; for example, individuals with major psychosis (originally thought to have severe personality disorder) and predatory sex

Table 3–2.   DSM-III Axis II disorders: SCID-II

	Number of participants	Percent
Borderline	178	69
Antisocial	142	55
Narcissistic	124	48
Paranoid	121	47
Passive-aggressive	81	31
Histrionic	64	25
Schizotypal	61	24
Avoidant	57	22
Dependent	52	20
Schizoid	30	12
Compulsive	26	10
Self-defeating	18	7
Psychopath (PCL-R 30 +)	100	39
No Axis II	10	4

Note.   Total sample size $N = 260$.

offenders who had committed particularly serious offenses; for example, one middle-class, middle-age, previously married pedophile had sadistic masturbatory offenses and had strangled a child. Male prisoners (who were the most severely behaviorally disturbed at the time of the study) received more diagnostic categories than the male and female participants detained in the maximum security hospitals. Borderline and avoidant personality disorders were more prevalent in the female participants, whereas antisocial, paranoid, passive-aggressive, histrionic, and narcissistic categories were more prevalent in the male prisoners. Male participants detained under the English legal category "Psychopathic disorder" demonstrated less Axis II comorbidity than the other two subsamples, with Narcissistic and Borderline categories most prevalent.

DSM-III Lifetime Axis I Mental Disorder

Half of all participants had at some time experienced a major depressive illness and more than one-third had been alcoholic or experienced serious problems due to alcohol abuse (see Table 3–3). Approximately one-fifth of the sample had suffered from dysthymia, phobias, unspecified psychotic episodes, drug dependence/abuse, or schizophrenia/schizophreniform disorders. A subgroup had never suffered from any Axis II disorder. The overall mean was 2.7 (SD, 1.9) lifetime diagnoses. This was reflected in the finding that more than half (132; 51%) had previously been inpatients in psychiatric hospitals, and 59 (23%) had at some time been treated with electroconvulsive therapy. In addition, 128 (49%) had at some time been prescribed antidepressant medication.

The female participants experienced considerably more Axis I psychopathology over the lifetime, in particular episodes of depression and mania/atypical bipolar disorder, unspecified psychotic episodes, phobias, anorexia nervosa, and gender identity disturbance. Deliberate self-harm was common in the overall sample, with 129 (50%) participants having a history of deliberate drug overdose and 151 (58%) a history of self-mutilation. These

---

Table 3-3.   Lifetime DSM-III Axis I disorder

	Number of participants	Percent
Depression	131	50
Alcoholism/abuse	95	37
Drug dependence/abuse	72	28
Dysthymia	59	23
Schizophrenia	58	22
Phobia	53	20
Unspecified psychosis	50	19
Panic/anxiety	47	18
Mania	38	15
Obsessive-compulsive	32	12
Transsexualism	27	10
Somatization	17	7
Delusional disorder	9	4
Anorexia nervosa	8	3
No Axis I	34	13

Note.   Total sample size $N = 260$.

behaviors were particularly common in the female participants, where 74 (80%) had taken drug overdoses and 85 (91%) had mutilated themselves.

Sexual Deviation

Sexual deviations were most common among the male participants in Broadmoor maximum security hospital, where 22 (26%) demonstrated sexual sadism; 15 (17%), pedophilia; 10 (12%), transvestism; 6 (7%), fetishism; 5 (65%), sexual masochism; 3 (4%), zoophilia; and 3 (4%), a history of exhibitionism. These categories showed comorbidity in certain individuals. The male prisoners showed relatively few paraphilias, as did the female prisoners, except in the case of 11 (12%) females with sexual sadism, usually involving sadomasochistic lesbian practices. Two women admitted being sexually attracted to children. Among the total sample, 31 (12%) participants described themselves as having a primary homosexual orientation, but an additional 59 (23%) described themselves as bisexual. There were no significant differences among subsamples. Overall, 36 (14%)

participants, of which 23 were female, admitted to a history of prostitution.

A total of 76 (29%) participants had at some time acted out (in their criminal history or undetected) sadistic masturbatory fantasies of rape or torture, masturbatory fantasies of homicide, or compulsive homicidal urges. Compulsive homicidal urges were more frequent in the female participants (23, 25%) than either sadistic masturbatory fantasies (2, 2%) or masturbation to fantasies of homicide (9, 10%). Nine (11%) male participants in Broadmoor maximum security hospital admitted to other sadistic (mainly rape) fantasies, a further 14 (15%) masturbated to fantasies of homicide, and 11 (13%) had experienced intermittent homicidal compulsions. Among the male prisoners, only 2 individuals admitted to sadistic fantasies, one of which included raping female children (which had resulted in an earlier conviction). The other masturbated to thoughts of homicide, which had culminated in the murder of a casual homosexual partner. However, 12 (15%) experienced intermittent overwhelming homicidal urges. It appeared that these urges were partly motivated by a pleasurable sense of power, exhilaration or excitement, and/or for the relief of tension and dysphoria.

Index Offenses

The majority of male and female participants were detained in maximum security hospitals under a hospital order with restrictions on discharge according to the English Mental Health Act, 1983, because they were considered a danger to the public. Two-thirds of the male prisoners were serving life sentences, reflecting the serious nature of their offending. Table 3–4 indicates that the criminal behavior of the overall sample mainly involved serious violence against the person. The subsample of male prisoners had more frequently been involved in acquisitive offenses and armed robberies; the male patients in Broadmoor Hospital had more frequently been involved in sexual offenses; and the females, in arson and property damage. Fewer females had been involved in personal violence. The motivation for homicide and

Table 3–4.   Index offenses

	Number of participants	Percent
Homicide	74	29
Attempted murder, wounding	74	29
Arson	59	23
Robbery, aggravated burglary	48	19
Assault, threats to kill	45	17
Theft	33	13
Rape, buggery, indecent assault	29	11
Property damage	23	9
Kidnap	8	3
Fraud	3	1
Blackmail	1	1
Non-crime admission	5	2

Note.   Total sample size N = 260.

serious violence among the male maximum security hospital patients was often of a sexual nature. The homicides and attempted murders of the overall sample also bore little resemblance to the usual U.K. picture of domestic killings or killings in the course of a quarrel, often when intoxicated (Mitchell 1990). Among the series were multiple killers, and the victims of some participants had been tortured and sexually abused. Sadistic violence in the overall sample was, as just indicated, by no means exclusively male.

Motivation

Table 3–5 lists the motivating factors for the participants' offenses. The defining characteristics of these variables are described in this chapter's appendix. A subgroup of 17 (7%) persons were considered to have been psychotic at the time of the index offense. In some cases, this had been during a relatively brief period of illness, usually schizophreniform disorder, from which the subject subsequently recovered. In others, there had been considerable uncertainty regarding the motivation of the offense at the time, and it had subsequently become clear as the subject's mental state had deteriorated that the offense had been

Table 3–5. Motivations for index offenses

Motivating factors	Number of participants (%)
Expressive aggression	31 (12)
Power, domination, control	47 (18)
Sexual gratification	45 (17)
Sadistic sexual fantasy	32 (12)
Paraphilia	15 (6)
Sexual conflict/trauma	8 (3)
Compulsive homicidal urge	53 (20)
Relief tension, dysphoria	82 (32)
Hyperirritability	67 (26)
Excitement exhilaration	51 (20)
Blow to self-esteem	30 (12)
Threat/actual loss	19 (7)
Psychotic	17 (7)
Intoxication	35 (14)
Revenge	49 (19)
Jealousy	14 (5)
Displaced aggression	65 (25)
Resolve problem/attention	33 (13)
Financial gain	67 (26)
Gang/group activity	36 (14)
Escape arrest	12 (5)
Pyromania	26 (10)
Undercontrolled aggression/fight	34 (13)
Victim precipitation/provocation	9 (4)

motivated by symptoms such as delusional beliefs. (The original intention in selecting this sample had been to exclude people with a primary diagnosis of major mental illness.)

Offenses of attempted murder, wounding, and grievous bodily harm demonstrated a statistical association with psychotic motivation (see Table 3–6). Offenses of homicide were associated with compulsive homicidal urges or urges to harm others, sexual conflict, victim precipitation, blows to the subject's self-esteem, and jealousy. As expected, serious offenses of rape, buggery, and indecent assault were associated with motivations of power, dominance, and obtaining control over the victim, expressive violence, the acting out of sadistic masturbatory fantasies, for the purpose of sexual gratification (including the acting out of paraphilias), and they were accompanied by the relief of tension and dysphoria. Table 3–6 also demonstrates that kidnap, usually of a child or young female, was associated with expres-

Table 3–6. Motivation for violent and sexual offenses, property damage, and acquisitive offending

Index offense	Motivation	Odds ratio	CI	Significance
Homicide	Compulsive homicidal urge	2.12	(1.13–3.97)	0.020
	Sexual conflict	4.42	(1.03–19.00)	0.030
	Victim precipitation	9.61	(1.95–47.43)	0.001
	Blow to self-esteem	2.48	(1.14–5.38)	0.020
	Jealousy	3.63	(1.21–10.87)	0.014
Attempted murder, wounding, grievous bodily harm	Psychotic	3.08	(1.14–8.32)	0.021
Rape, buggery, indecent assault	Power, domination, control	9.49	(4.13–21.84)	0.000
	Expressive violence	9.61	(4.00–23.08)	0.000
	Sadistic fantasy	5.00	(2.07–12.09)	0.000
	Sexual gratification	18.31	(7.52–44.56)	0.000
	Paraphilia	12.19	(4.02–36.94)	0.000
	Relief tension, dysphoria	2.96	(1.63–5.40)	0.000
Kidnap	Expressive violence	8.33	(1.97–35.25)	0.001
	Sexual gratification	8.83	(2.03–38.44)	0.001
	Sadistic fantasy	4.61	(1.05–20.32)	0.030
Arson	Revenge	4.83	(2.47–9.41)	0.000
	Displaced aggression	4.43	(2.37–8.28)	0.000
	Excitement/exhilaration	3.53	(1.83–6.81)	0.000
	Force problem resolution	7.42	(3.40–16.16)	0.000
	Pyromania	68.23	(15.63–301.70)	0.000
Property damage	Undercontrolled aggression	3.40	(1.28–9.02)	0.010
	Excitement/exhilaration	3.68	(1.51–8.96)	0.003
Theft	Financial gain	5.06	(2.37–10.83)	0.000
Robbery, aggravated burglary	Financial gain	67.37	(24.32–186.61)	0.000
	Gang/group activity	10.51	(3.97–27.82)	0.000
Firearm	Financial gain	10.85	(3.77–31.23)	0.000
	Escape arrest	16.71	(4.77–58.54)	0.000

Note. Total sample size $N = 260$; CI = confidence interval.

sive violence, sexual gratification, and acting out sadistic fantasies.

Offenses of arson were characterized by a range of different motivations, including revenge, displaced aggression, and (nonsexual) excitement, or were designed to force others to resolve the offender's problems or drew attention to them. It was unsurprising that pyromania motivated many of these offenses. However, the presence of a substantial number of (mainly female) participants with pyromania does indicate the unusual and highly selected nature of the sample.

Property damage was considerably more frequent in female participants and was associated with excitement, exhilaration, and uncontrolled aggression. It was unsurprising that offenses of theft, robbery, and aggravated burglary were carried out for financial gain and that, in a subgroup of these offenses, robbery and aggravated burglary were often a gang or group activity, sometimes carried out with firearms, which were used to evade arrest.

Table 3–7 demonstrates the independent associations between index offenses and Axis II and lifetime Axis I psychopathology. This table also reflects the specific qualities of an unusual sample who had committed very serious crimes and who were considered a grave danger to the public. In this sample, offenses of homicide were associated with narcissistic personality disorder, attempted murder, wounding, and grievous bodily harm with paranoid personality disorders, and arson with borderline personality disorder. Acquisitive offenses such as robbery, firearm offenses, and theft were associated with antisocial personality disorder.

Lifetime Axis I Disorders and Criminal Motivation

Table 3–8 demonstrates the independent associations between motivating factors and Axis I disorders present over the lifetime after controlling for potential confounding from comorbid Axis I disorders and Axis II categories, using logistic regression. As expected, diagnoses of schizophrenia and delusional disorder

Table 3–7. Association between index offenses and psychopathology

Index offense	Diagnostic category	Odds ratio	CI	Significance
Homicide	Narcissistic	2.27	(1.31–3.95)	0.003
	Panic/anxiety[a]	2.18	(1.13–4.20)	0.018
Attempted murder, wounding	Paranoid	1.92	(1.11–3.32)	0.018
Arson	Borderline	12.09	(3.65–39.45)	0.000
Property damage	Obsessive-compulsive[a]	2.86	(1.04–7.91)	0.035
Robbery	Antisocial	5.39	(2.41–12.10)	0.000
Firearm	Antisocial	5.21	(1.49–18.26)	0.005
Theft	Antisocial	3.87	(1.49–7.69)	0.005
	Histrionic	3.03	(1.40–6.54)	0.005
Kidnap	Schizoid	5.00	(1.13–22.09)	0.020

Note. Total sample size $N = 260$; CI = confidence interval.
[a] Lifetime Axis I disorder.

Table 3–8. Associations between motivations for index offenses and lifetime Axis I disorders

Axis I category	Motivation	Adjusted odds ratio	CI	Significance
Schizophrenia	Psychotic	14.30	(4.45–49.91)	0.000
Delusional disorder	Psychotic	14.64	(3.51–61.10)	0.000
	Jealousy	10.91	(2.41–49.48)	0.000
Dysthymia	Loss	3.81	(1.43–10.07)	0.007
Alcoholism/abuse	Intoxication	4.31	(1.90–9.67)	0.001
Drug dependence/abuse	Intoxication	2.59	(1.19–5.61)	0.020
Unspecified psychosis	Excitement/exhilaration	2.18	(1.07–4.39)	0.031
Obsessive-compulsive	Compulsive homicidal urge	7.50	(3.33–16.84)	0.000
	Relief tension, dysphoria	3.91	(1.67–9.11)	0.002
Anorexia nervosa	Resolve problem	7.69	(1.82–32.41)	0.001
Transsexualism	Resolve problem	3.22	(1.28–8.08)	0.013
	Pyromania	4.20	(1.61–10.80)	0.003

Total sample size $N = 260$; CI = confidence interval

were associated with psychotic motivation at the time of the offense. Similarly, delusional disorder was associated with morbid jealousy. Alcoholism/alcohol abuse and drug dependence/abuse were associated with intoxication at the time of the offense. Individuals with a lifetime history of dysthymia were more likely to commit offenses precipitated by loss. Those with lifetime anorexia nervosa and transsexualism offended in an attempt to resolve problems or attract attention to themselves or their situation. Participants with transsexualism were also more likely to set fires as a result of pyromania. Obsessive-compulsive disorder was associated with violent offenses that had been preceded by repetitive compulsive urges to harm or to kill others and offenses that were intended to result in the relief of symptoms of tension and/or dysphoria. Participants who had experienced brief psychotic episodes were more likely to commit offenses for the purpose of experiencing excitement and exhilaration. No independent associations were found between the motivations in Table 3–5 and lifetime diagnoses of depressive disorder, phobic disorder, panic/anxiety disorder, mania/atypical bipolar disorder, or somatization disorder.

Axis II Disorders and Criminal Motivation

In cluster A, paranoid personality disorder was independently associated with offenses characterized by undercontrolled aggression and those motivated by revenge (see Table 3–9). Schizoid personality disorder was associated with expressive aggression and offenses carried out for excitement/exhilaration. No associations were found between any motivational variables included in the study and schizotypal personality disorder.

Cluster C compulsive personality disorder was independently associated with offenses that were preceded by hyperirritability in the offender, displaced aggression, and the experience of loss or threatened loss. No associations were found between the motivational variables and avoidant or dependent, or with the other personality disorders not included in any cluster, such as passive-aggressive and self-defeating personality disorders.

There were several observed associations between the cluster B personality disorders and motivational variables included in the study. Antisocial personality associated with hyperirritability, offenses carried out for financial gain, and offenses carried out in a gang or as a group activity. Histrionic personality disorder was also associated with offenses carried out for financial gain and behavior intended to avoid arrest or detection. Narcissistic personality disorder was associated with offenses motivated by the need for power, domination, and control of a victim and by blows to the subject's self-esteem. Borderline personality disorder was associated with multiple motivational variables, including compulsive homicidal urges/urges to harm, relief of tension/dysphoria, hyperirritability, revenge, displaced aggression, excitement/exhilaration, desire to resolve problems, and pyromania. In this sample, all individuals with pyromania had a diagnosis of borderline personality disorder.

Discussion

Methodological Considerations

The high prevalence of lifetime Axis I and Axis II psychopathology found in the study is likely to reflect the unusual nature of the sample. This reflected referred individuals who were accepted for admission to English maximum security hospitals and a group of prisoners who were so disruptive and dangerous that they had been placed in special units for their management. In terms of abnormality of personality, antisocial behavior, and risk of serious harm to the public, this sample was at the far end of the spectrum of severity for the entire population of England and Wales. Nevertheless, in the absence of adequate, epidemiologically based data on the associations between diagnostic categories and criminal behavior, the extent to which this sample truly deviated or showed particularly unusual patterns of association compared with other serious offenders must remain uncertain. Certain associations were as expected, such as those between lifetime diagnoses of substance abuse and intoxication while of-

Table 3–9. Association between motivations for index offenses and clusters A, B, and C DSM-III Axis II disorders

Axis II category	Motivation	Adjusted odds ratio	CI	Significance
Cluster A				
Paranoid	Undercontrolled aggression	2.73	(1.26–5.86)	0.010
	Revenge	2.88	(1.49–5.56)	0.001
Schizoid	Expressive aggression	2.79	(1.08–7.18)	0.034
	Excitement/exhilaration	2.75	(1.21–6.25)	0.012
Schizotypal	—	—	—	—
Cluster C				
Compulsive	Hyperirritability	1.99	(1.06–3.74)	0.030
	Displaced aggression	2.93	(1.28–6.71)	0.009
	Loss	4.21	(1.37–12.67)	0.011
Avoidant	—	—	—	—
Dependent	—	—	—	—
Other				
Passive aggressive	—	—	—	—
Self-defeating	—	—	—	—

Cluster B

					p
Antisocial	Hyperirritability	3.17	(1.67–5.98)		0.000
	Financial gain	5.10	(2.44–10.48)		0.000
Borderline	Gang/group activity	4.07	(1.71–9.67)		0.001
	Compulsive homicidal urge	3.23	(2.95–7.74)		0.009
	Relief tension, dysphoria	14.36	(4.99–41.26)		0.000
	Hyperirritability	2.46	(1.18–5.05)		0.000
	Revenge	2.77	(1.23–6.21)		0.011
	Displaced aggression	1.95	(1.01–3.78)		0.045
	Excitement/exhilaration	3.78	(1.52–9.29)		0.004
	Resolve problem	4.35	(1.27–14.87)		0.020
	Pyromania	$			0.000
Histrionic	Financial gain	2.23	(1.13–4.06)		0.019
	Avoid arrest	4.05	(1.20–13.32)		0.023
Narcissistic	Power, domination, control	2.23	(1.16–4.29)		0.014
	Blow to self-esteem	4.05	(2.45–17.90)		0.000

Note. Total sample size $N = 260$. $ = stable odds ratio not obtained due to small cell size. CI = confidence interval.

fending, and antisocial personality disorder and offending for financial gain, and appeared to support the validity of the findings. Furthermore, the severity and range of psychopathology that had resulted in multiple diagnostic categories, and a range of serious crimes with complex and multiple motivations, may well have resulted in increased statistical power to determine these associations.

The most serious limitations of the study include the involvement of only one researcher in eliciting both the diagnostic information and the data on the criminal behavior. This could have increased the probability of confirming any associations that might have been expected by the researcher. However, resource limitations precluded the involvement of a second researcher.

Axis II Categories and Criminal Motivation

The study has demonstrated that Axis II categories, in certain circumstances, appear to make a substantial contribution to the motivation of serious criminal behavior. However, the confirmation of some of these statistical associations would require additional data and would need to exclude the possibility of confounded associations due to other factors that were simply not measured. Nevertheless, many of the findings confirmed the expected relationship between Axis II disorders and behavior.

Antisocial Personality Disorder

In this sample, crimes involving financial gain, including thefts, robberies, and firearm offenses, were associated with antisocial personality disorder (ASPD). ASPD is a pervasive pattern of disregard for, and violation of, the rights of others that begins in childhood or early adolescence and continues into adulthood. Successive DSM classifications have moved closer to the current ICD-10 category dissocial personality disorder, and an attempt has been made to include the abnormal personality traits considered to be associated with this condition rather than a diagnostic construct that is predominantly defined by behavioral disorder. However, the DSM-III category used in this study was largely determined by behaviors. It has previously been observed that ASPD shows considerable overlap with the criminological construct of the career criminal (Coid 1993a; Dolan and Coid 1993; Farrington 1995). In this sample, persons with ASPD were characterized by having more extensive previous histories of acquisitive offending than other participants, and many individuals were associated with criminal organizations and other professional criminals.

A subgroup of ASPD participants had been involved in crimes of violence. Furthermore, violence had characterized many of the acquisitive crimes for which they had been convicted. In some of these cases, the offense had been preceded by intense irritability in the subject, and the outburst had been precipitated by minimal provocation, correlating with criterion (4) of the DSM-IV construct "irritability and aggressiveness, as indicated by repeated physical fights or assaults."

Case 1. Axis II: Antisocial, Narcissistic

A 22-year-old man with a history of acquisitive offending since the age of 13 was sentenced to 18 years imprisonment for nine offenses of robbery, two of grievous bodily harm, and possession of firearms. He had been convicted along with five other persons and was believed to be the leader of a gang of criminals who had been involved in a series of armed robberies. In one robbery, he had shot a passerby in the face with a sawn-off shotgun and in another, during the course of a getaway, had shot a taxi driver in the back. In prison his behavior was highly disruptive, and he spent long periods in solitary confinement following assaults on prison officers and damage to prison property. He looked younger than his age and prison staff believed that his behavior was often designed to gain status in the eyes of his fellow prisoners as well as due to a low threshold for violent behavior when his wishes were not complied with.

Borderline Personality Disorder

The range of associations observed between borderline personality disorder (BPD) and motivations for offending are of considerable interest and indicate the complexity of the associations between BPD and crime. BPD characterized the majority of female participants and was strongly related to offenses of arson, committed primarily by females in this sample. All cases of arson due to pyromania were in participants with BPD. It must be questioned to what extent the impulse disorder constituted a condition that was truly distinct from BPD. Although BPD is considered an Axis II disorder, this view is not shared by all commentators (Akiskal 1992; Akiskal and Akiskal 1992; Coid 1993b). The "hybrid" quality of BPD psychopathology has also been observed, specifically the combination of abnormal personality traits and mood disorder. In a previous study of the female participants, behaviors such as fire setting, self-mutilation, binge eating, property damage, assaults against the person, and compulsive homicidal urges were found to be directly associated with brief mood swings. The intense affective symptoms associated with these mood disturbances appeared to have a direct influence on the women's behavior. Participants reported relief and the reduction of the intensity of these symptoms as an outcome of these behaviors, many of which were carried out deliberately for this purpose, and where one behavior could be substituted for another (Coid 1993b).

Case 2. Axis II: Borderline, Narcissistic, Histrionic, Dependent. Lifetime Axis I: Depressive Disorder, Somatization, Pyromania

A 30-year-old woman was convicted of arson after setting fire to a kiosk where sweets and tobacco were sold. She had a history of depression dating from her midteens and had begun to take repeated overdoses of medication, which resulted in frequent hospitalization. She frequently self-mutilated and in her late teens began to make hoax telephone calls to the police and fire brigade. After her mother's death, her periods of hospitalization became longer, and attempts to rehabilitate her resulted in further overdoses or other behavior that prevented her discharge. After a further attempt at rehabilitation to a hostel, she attempted to break into the kiosk. After her release from police custody, she returned and set fire in revenge for the shopkeeper reporting her. After compulsory admission to a psychiatric hospital, there was a further deterioration in her behavior; she set 14 fires in separate incidents before being transferred to a maximum security hospital. She described compulsory thoughts of killing others by setting fires and admitted that she was fascinated by fire and excited by the sound of sirens. She described the experience of fire setting, and then watching the flames, as relieving her mood swings, which were characterized by symptoms of severe dysphoria and tension. The achievement of setting a large fire was sexually arousing to her, sometimes to the point of orgasm. Treatment with neuroleptics was of moderate benefit in helping her to control her urges.

A model that postulates that impulsive behavior occurs in response to dysphoric affect in BPD, to account for criminal behavior, contrasts with the conventional explanation of the association between impulsive behaviors and personality traits embodied in the DSM-IV construct. According to the traditional view, the criminal act would be perceived as the outcome of generalized instability in interpersonal relationships, self-image, affects, and impulse control in the subject. Thus, motivations of displaced aggression and hyperirritability might be considered the outcome of criterion (8) of BPD "inappropriate, intense anger, or difficulty controlling anger," and revenge of criterion (9) "transient, stress-related paranoid ideation," or alternatively criterion (2) "a pattern of unstable and intense interpersonal relationships characterized by alternating between extremes of idealization and devaluation." Similarly, criminal behavior carried out to force others to resolve the subject's problems or to draw attention to the offender's situation could correlate with criterion (1) "frantic efforts to avoid real or imagined abandonment." Furthermore, the potentially self-damaging impulsivity of patients with borderline disorder (criterion 4) could also, in certain persons, have been motivated by a desire for exhilaration and excitement.

Case 3. Axis II: Antisocial, Borderline, Paranoid,
Histrionic. Lifetime Axis I Depressive Disorder: Alcohol
Dependency, Drug Abuse

A 22-year-old woman with a history of conduct disorder, substance abuse, and frequent criminal convictions in her late teens and early adulthood, including assault and possession of bladed weapons, had been admitted to a psychiatric hospital for the treatment of a depressive episode. She had formed a relationship with a male patient but subsequently discovered that he had been seeing another female patient. She entered the dormitory where she believed her rival was sleeping, removed her bedclothes, and stabbed her several times with a knife she had obtained from the hospital kitchens and had specially sharpened. Realizing that the person she had stabbed was the wrong person, she continued to stab her victim because she enjoyed the pleasurable sensation that stabbing gave her. She was highly assaultive to staff and other patients after transfer into maximum security and described mood swings and extreme hyperirritability, but also enjoyment from being physically restrained by the nursing staff during her violent outbursts.

Histrionic Personality Disorder

Histrionic personality disorder was more prevalent in the male prisoner subsample, many of whom were professional criminals. This group had the highest scores on Hare's Psychopathy Checklist (Hare 1991), indicating a combination of career criminality and psychopathy, thus explaining the statistical association with acquisitive crime, motivations of financial gain, and avoiding arrest. It is probable that these participants' overly dramatic, reactive, and intensely expressed behavior, together with characteristic disturbances in their interpersonal relationships due to their shallowness, egocentricity, and vain and demanding behavior, overlapped substantially with PCL-R criteria of glibness, superficial charm, grandiose sense of self-worth, shallow affect, and callousness.

Narcissistic Personality Disorder

The association between narcissistic personality disorder (NPD) and crimes motivated by the need for power, domination, and control, and precipitated by a blow to the offender's self-esteem, are entirely consistent with the psychodynamic literature on narcissistic personality organization. DSM-IV defines NPD as a pervasive pattern of grandiosity, need for admiration, and lack of empathy that begins in early childhood and is present in a variety of contexts. However, the DSM construct fails to describe the dynamic interaction between the various components of pathological narcissism and certain covert characteristics, such as the inordinate hypersensitivity; the feelings of inferiority and worthlessness, which are concealed behind narcissistic individuals' inflated self-regard and grandiosity; and the intense envy behind their contempt and devaluation of others (Akhtar and Thompson 1982). Offenses carried out to satisfy needs for power, domination, and control (in the majority of cases involving serious sexual assaults on females) clearly fulfilled their narcissistic grandiosity and the need to be superior, together with their ruthless exploitation, egocentricity, sense of entitlement, and lack of empathy while carrying out the criminal act. But behind these overt feelings of disturbed self-concept were often lifelong feelings of inferiority, worthlessness, and fragility. In these participants, the DSM-III NPD construct may not have been adequate to describe the lower-level psychopathology of these individuals, many of whom demonstrated malignant narcissism or qualities of the "antisocial proper" described by Kernberg (1984).

A proportion of the homicides in this series were carried out by narcissistic individuals in a state of "narcissistic rage." The specific qualities of anger and violence in relation to NPD have been described by Kohut (1973) as a profoundly angry reaction to injury to self-esteem, in which there is an accompanying need for revenge and the undoing of hurt by whatever means is necessary. The individual shows a compulsion in the pursuit of revenge with total disregard for reasonable limits of behavior. The irrationality of the vengeful attitude is particularly frightening, and the individual may retain not only an intact but also a sharpened capacity for reasoning, despite the intensity of affect. These factors lead to the ruthless completion of the act despite its irrationality and the ultimate cost to the individual and society. Rosen (1989, 1991) has drawn attention to the importance of faulty regulation of self-esteem in narcissistic individuals, who may resort to any means to redress the balance, including physical action and aggression, sexual stimulation, substance abuse, or risk-taking.

Case 4. Axis II: Narcissistic

A 25-year-old male was convicted of manslaughter and after a short prison sentence was released on parole. He had a history of repeated difficulties in his relationships with women in which he would typically choose a promiscuous partner, but then behave in a violent manner toward her, or else he would disappear for a week at a time when a partner's affection grew for him, thereby distancing her from him and sometimes resulting in the woman forming relationships with other men. However, these new relationships would lead to jealousy and further violence in retaliation from the subject. The index offense occurred following a telephone call to his former cohabitee, when he asked for the return of some of his belongings from their apartment. During the telephone conversation, the subject became increasingly angry and jealous when he realized that her new boyfriend was present. He petulantly insisted that she should give his sweater that he had left behind, and which he had received from her as a Christmas present, to her new boyfriend. Unfortunately, his ex-girlfriend's mother was listening on the telephone extension and at that point interrupted and informed him that there would be little point in giving it to the new boyfriend, because he was considerably larger in physique and the sweater would be too small. His immediate reaction of rage was so extreme that he put down the telephone, walked to a shop where he deliberately purchased a butcher's knife, then traveled by bus to his girlfriend's apartment with the deliberate intention of killing her. After kicking open the door, he was confronted by the boyfriend whom he stabbed to death instead, subsequently claiming that he had acted in self-defense. This was successfully argued on his behalf by his lawyer when he appeared in court.

Paranoid Personality Disorder

Paranoid personality disorder demonstrated a high prevalence in this sample, which is in contrast to community studies and previously described clinic samples. In these participants, paranoid personality was strongly comorbid with ASPD. It appeared that the paranoid, sensitive, and vengeful traits of many of these individuals added an additional dimension of potential dangerousness to their already criminal disposition, thereby exacerbating their ready tendency to get involved in fights, and as a result of minimal provocation. Sometimes the offenses were motivated by revenge for real or imagined slights.

Schizoid Personality Disorder

In this sample, schizoid personality appeared to correspond to the syndrome described by Wolff and Chick (1980) based on the developmental observation of a group of emotionally withdrawn and socially detached children, some participants presenting features of Asperger's syndrome (Wing 1983). These individuals had a history of neurodevelopmental disorder and tended to come from families of a higher social class than the rest of the sample. They had an absence of a history of mental disorder and criminality in their family, but a high prevalence of obstetric complications and early developmental delay. Their offending behavior was not motivated by obvious external precipitants and had often involved the acting out of fantasies or sexual deviations that were associated with comorbid paraphilias. Additional qualities of these offenses involved excitement and exhilaration and the use of expressive violence. These offenses had sometimes been unexpected, and overt aggression had often been entirely absent from the offenders' criminal histories.

Case 5. Axis II: Schizoid, Schizotypal

A 9-year-old girl's body was found in a wooded area having been stabbed 39 times in the chest, back, and neck. Seven years later, a 22-year-old man was arrested after acting suspiciously in the same location. He was wearing rubber gloves and in possession of a large sheath knife, a strip of adhesive tape, and rope. Under interrogation he admitted to the first killing and that he was looking for a second victim. He had worked as a bookkeeper in a firm of accountants where his record had been exemplary. He had no previous convictions. He had been socially withdrawn and friendless since early childhood and had never had a girlfriend. He lived at home with his father and stepmother, where he would spend his time alone, watching television in his room or reading violent pornography. He admitted to having fantasies of killing women since the age of 12 years. These had become increasingly intrusive and compulsive but had subsided after the homicide, for which he had evaded detection, when aged 15. They had reemerged 1 year before his arrest. His demeanor at interview was strikingly cold and unemotional. He denied sexual arousal during his crimes or a desire to have sex.

Compulsive Personality Disorder

Compulsive personality disorder was defined in DSM-III as a category in which there is generally a restricted ability to express warm and tender emotions, perfectionism that interferes with the ability to grasp the "big picture," insistence that others submit to his or her way of doing things, obsessive devotion to work or productivity to the exclusion of pleasure, and indecisiveness.

Loss or threatened loss may be particularly difficult to cope with in a personality characterized by rigid and inflexible traits. However, the higher functioning qualities of these traits may also result in these individuals displacing their resulting anger onto inanimate objects or other persons less valued than the original provoking agent.

Future Research

This chapter has confirmed the importance of the Axis II diagnostic categories in the forensic assessment of serious offenders and indicates that the arguments of Widiger and Trull (1994) are premature in suggesting that there should be a major shift to a dimensional model. Nevertheless, future research may require dimensional models to explore the relationship between personality traits and more common and less serious criminal behaviors. Crime is highly prevalent in society, and it is unlikely that most crimes are related to specific Axis II categories. However, dimensional scores could still be derived from the current Axis II categorization for use in the study of less serious criminal behavior.

The taxonomy used in this study is clearly a prototype and requires further refinement, followed by studies designed to test its reliability and validity. However, despite the unidimensional nature of its descriptive properties, and the compression of its time span to cover only the immediate period before and during the commission of the offense, it does provide a potential basis on which to develop more detailed routine assessments of serious offenders. Future developments might employ a more complex longitudinal approach to criminal behavior based on that described by Ressler et al. (1988). But whether the associations that can be established between patterns of offending and personality disorder categories will ultimately prove helpful in future criminal investigations remains unclear. Ressler et al. (1988) described the profile characteristics and crime scene differences between "organized" and "disorganized" murders. Many of these characteristics have clear correlations with certain personality traits, but these associations remain as yet untested. However, future study of the contribution of abnormal personality to the risk of reoffending is clearly of major importance in determining the release of offenders back into the community. High scores on traits of narcissism may well indicate an increased risk of extreme violence in the future, following a similar blow to the individual's self-esteem. Similarly, high scores on criteria for paranoid personality may indicate an increased risk of explosive violence following minimal provocation, especially in the presence of ASPD. However, the major challenge within this area of future research is to resolve the difficulties in predicting exactly which situational factors are important in precipitating reoffending in combination with and in the context of specific dispositional factors of Axis II psychopathology.

Appendix: Taxonomy of Motivation

The taxonomic system used in this study evolved inductively. A similar process has been employed by Toch et al. (1989) in classifying the manipulative behaviors of prison inmates. The aim was to separate 1) the various elements that had motivated a criminal act immediately prior, including goals that the behavior was intending to achieve, and 2) additional key factors that had shaped the behavior, such as intoxication, the presence of others, and so on. The variables included in the taxonomy were derived from previous observations from clinical practice and from the research literature, including established classifications of criminal behavior based on motivation rather than characteristics of the actions themselves. The taxonomy was not based on the type of victim, location, and so on, although these factors could clearly still have a bearing on the determination of the offender's motivation.

The intention of the proposed taxonomy was not to include mutually exclusive categories, as different motivations can exist simultaneously. Furthermore, additional modifying factors can arise while an offense is being carried out.

Case 6. Axis II: Antisocial, Narcissistic. Lifetime Axis I: Pedophilia, Sexual Sadism

A 17-year-old male with a previous conviction of indecent assault on a 4-year-old boy was convicted of attempted murder of a 15-year-old boy. He himself had been molested and raped by an adult neighbor when aged 14 and had subsequently engaged in homosexual activities with boys of a similar age or younger. His masturbatory fantasies had increasingly involved the tying up, humiliation, and beating of boys prior to the index offense. He had finally lured a 15-year-old to a disused building with the intention of raping him. He grabbed the boy from behind in a neck lock and ordered him to remove his trousers. When the child refused, he strangled him to unconsciousness and tore off his clothing. He then changed his mind about his originally intended sexual assault and decided to ensure that the boy was dead by strangling him, then tying his trouser legs tightly around his neck, subsequently concealing the body. The boy regained consciousness, and the police were notified.

In this example, the offender admitted to an overwhelming urge for sexual gratification on first encountering his victim. It had been established by the time of interview that his primary sexual orientation was to prepubertal and adolescent boys. Prior to offense, there had been a progressive escalation in the sadistic component of his masturbatory fantasies. It continued to remain unclear whether these had developed and progressed to include a homicidal climax, or whether the lifeless form of his victim had, as he told the police, resulted in a diminution of his level of sexual arousal. Nevertheless, he admitted that his subsequent determination to kill had been motivated for the purpose of escaping arrest. For this offense the motivations coded according to Table 3–5 included sexual gratification, sadistic sexual fantasy, paraphilia, and escape arrest. Table 3–5 has already listed the motivations and modifying factors involved in the index offenses of the sample of 260 participants. These categories are defined as follows:

1. *Expressive aggression:* The offense is characterized by high expressive aggression (unprovoked physical and verbal aggression or physical force in excess of that necessary to gain victim compliance must be present). Rage is clearly evident in the offense. Typically seen in "anger" rape, as described by Groth and Birnbaum (1979) and Ressler et al. (1993), where the primary motivation for the offense is anger and not sexual gratification. There may be behaviors included under sadistic sexual fantasy, such as demeaning and humiliating the victim, but these are punishing actions done in anger and not to increase sexual arousal, as in that category. These offenses are predominantly impulse-driven (e.g., opportunity, possibly coupled with impaired judgment due drugs/alcohol). They often involve an element of displaced aggression, which compensates for an accumulation of real or imagined insults, humiliations from others.
2. *Power, domination, control:* The offense involves a need to achieve dominance and control over a victim. Typically observed in the "power–reassurance rapist," as described by Ressler et al. (1993), when the assault is primarily an expression of rape fantasies. There is often a history of sexual preoccupation, typified by having acted or fantasized a variety of perversions. There is often high sexual arousal accompanied by a loss of self-control, causing a distorted perception of the victim/offender relationship (e.g., the rapist may want the victim to respond in a sexual or erotic manner, may make a date for the future with the victim). The offender is usually compensating for acutely felt inadequacies.
3. *Sexual gratification:* The offense involves the gratification of sexual desire, including sexual deviations.
4. *Sadistic sexual fantasy:* The offense is the enactment or attempted enactment of a sadistic sexual fantasy. There must have been previous rehearsal in the offender's imagination that is reinforced by masturbation, as described by MacCulloch et al. (1983). The offense must be a "try-out" of the fantasy or the culmination of one or more previous "try-outs."
5. *Paraphilia:* The offense involves acting upon one or more paraphilias defined by DSM-IV as (a) recurrent, intense sexually arousing fantasies, sexual urges, or behaviors generally in-

volving (1) nonhuman objects, (2) the suffering or humiliation of oneself or one partner, or (3) children or other nonconsenting persons that occur over a period of at least 6 months; and (b) causing clinically significant distress or impairment in social, occupational, or other important areas of functioning.

6. *Sexual conflict:* These offenses are precipitated, rather than motivated, by unresolved conscious or subconscious conflicts resulting from earlier experiences. The behavior of the victim or circumstances may result in sudden, extreme anxiety to the extent of panic and/or extreme rage and, in most cases, relate to traumatic early experiences, typically sexual abuse.

Case 7. Axis II: Antisocial, Borderline, Narcissistic, Paranoid. Lifetime Axis I: Depressive Disorder, Schizophreniform Disorder, Alcohol and Drug Abuse

A 20-year-old male had failed to comply with the conditions of his parole and was on the run from the police. He had previously engaged in male prostitution and was picked up while hitchhiking by a middle-aged homosexual. After spending the night with the older man, he became enraged when the latter casually dismissed him the next morning, telling him to leave as soon as possible and make his own way to the nearest road. The offender described suddenly experiencing the same intense feelings of rage and humiliation as he typically felt with his stepfather, whom the victim physically resembled, and who had repeatedly sexually assaulted him during his adolescence. He beat the older man to death with a wooden mallet. (Sexual conflict and blow to self-esteem both coded.)

7. *Hyperirritability:* The offender describes being in a state of intense anger or irritability prior to the offense. The irritability preceded the encounter and had not been provoked by the victim. The victim may, in some cases, have behaved in a provocative manner, but the irritability preceded the provocation. The emotion of anger/irritability had arisen independently and constitutes an intense mood. There may have

been some minimal provocation or external stress prior to encountering the victim, but this factor must be distinguished from displaced aggression. The irritable, angry feelings have no clear focus or causation in the mind of the offender.

8. *Relief of tension/dysphoria:* The offense is preceded by intense feelings of anxiety, tension, anger and/or dysphoria prior to the act. These symptoms are relieved by the offending behavior. The offense is often carried out deliberately for this purpose. The same dynamic process is frequently seen in self-mutilation. The offender may describe interchanging several behaviors, including self-mutilation and criminal behavior, to relieve symptoms (see Coid 1993b; Coid et al. 1992).

9. *Excitement/exhilaration:* The offense is deliberately carried out for the purpose of pleasurable (nonsexual) excitement and/ or a feeling of exhilaration.

10. *Compulsive urge to harm/kill:* The offender describes compulsive urges to do physical harm to others. In certain cases this takes the form of urges to kill other persons. This urge cannot be explained by precipitating factors such as provocation or revenge and should not include offenses where there is any element of provocation or revenge. The offender may describe obsessive, intrusive thoughts and may attempt to resist these urges.

11. *Blow to self-esteem:* The offense is precipitated by words or actions by the victim, or potential victim, which resulted in a blow to the offender's self-esteem, resulting in feelings of humiliation, devaluation, and consequent rage. The self-esteem of these individuals is typically fragile and poorly regulated (see Rosen 1979, 1991), resulting in an extreme and sometimes prolonged reaction of rage.

12. *Threatened/actual loss:* The offense is precipitated by loss or threatened loss of another person, object, or a supportive situation, such as loss of accommodation. Loss typically provokes feelings of extreme anxiety, distress, and/or anger in the offender.

13. *Undercontrolled aggression:* The offender has a previous history of a low threshold for violence following minimal prov-

ocation. The offense often occurs following an altercation with another person, resulting in a fight.

14. *Victim precipitation:* Details of the offense include undisputed evidence that the victim provoked the behavior of the offender, usually offering aggression before the subject retaliated (this category is not applied to victims of sexual assault).

15. *Revenge:* The offense is carried out in retaliation for a perceived wrong, real, imagined, or delusional, committed against the offender or a significant other.

16. *Jealousy:* Jealousy can be coded in circumstances in which the individual has discovered true infidelity, where the jealousy is considered to be "morbid," and in cases where it is delusional.

17. *Displaced aggression:* The offense is committed on another person or object in place of the individual who originally provoked the reaction of anger in the offender. The offense may occur because the provoking agent or preferred victim is not available, may be more effectively able to defend themselves, or because the offender does not wish to harm the person who originally provoked the angry reaction.

18. *Problem resolution/attention seeking:* The offense is committed to draw attention to the plight of the offender, to persuade or force others to resolve the offender's problems, or to meet the needs of the offender for attention or care.

19. *Financial gain:* The offense is carried out with the intention and expectation of financial gain.

20. *Escape arrest:* The behavior is designed to avoid detection or escape arrest.

21. *Pyromania:* Fire setting is the outcome of a DSM-IV diagnosis of pyromania, defined as (a) deliberate and purposeful fire setting on more than one occasion, (b) tension or affective arousal before the act, (c) fascination with, interest in, curiosity about, or attraction to fire and its situation or context, (d) pleasure, gratification, or relief when setting fires, or when witnessing or participating in their aftermath, (e) not done for monetary gain, an expression of sociopolitical ideology, to conceal criminal activity, to express anger or vengeance, to improve living circumstances, in response to a

delusional hallucination, or as a result of impaired judgement (in dementia, mental retardation, substance intoxication), and (f) not better accounted for by conduct disorder, a manic episode, or antisocial personality disorder.

22. *Gang/group activity:* The offense is carried out by the offender within a group or as part of an organized gang.

23. *Intoxication:* This category combines intoxication due to both drugs and alcohol at the time of the offense.

24. *Psychotic:* The offense was directly motivated, or demonstrated substantial influence in its motivation, from symptoms of mental illness, including schizophrenia, schizoaffective disorder, mania, psychotic depression, or an unspecified psychotic episode.

25. *To be a hero:* The offender commits the offense in a manner that other persons or factors would be blamed, and in which he or she would take the credit for subsequent events; for example, apparently rescuing or attempting to rescue a victim, alerting the authorities, resuscitating the victim, and so on.

References

Akhtar S, Thomson JA: Overview: narcissistic personality disorder. Am J Psychiatry 139:12–20, 1982

Akiskal HS: Delineating irritable and hyperthymic variants of the cyclothymic temperament. Journal of Personality Disorders 6:326–342, 1992

Akiskal HS, Akiskal K: Cyclothymic, hyperthymic, and depressive temperaments as subaffective variants of mood disorders, in American Psychiatric Press Review of Psychiatry, Vol II. Edited by Tasman A, Riba MB. Washington, DC, American Psychiatric Press, 1992, pp 43–62

Amir M: Patterns in Forcible Rape. Chicago, IL, Chicago University Press, 1971

Blackburn R: Personality in relation to extreme aggression in psychiatric offenders. Br J Psychiatry 114:821–828, 1968

Blackburn R: Personality types among abnormal homicides. Br J Criminology 11:14–31, 1971

Blackburn R: An empirical classification of psychopathic personality. Br J Psychiatry 127:456–460, 1975

Blackburn R: Patterns of personality deviation among violent offenders. Br J Criminology 26:254–269, 1986

Blackburn R: Psychopathlogy and personality disorder in relation to violence, in Clinical Approaches to Violence. Edited by Howells K, Hollin CR. Chichester, Wiley, 1989, pp 61–87

Box S: Power, Crime, and Mystification. London, Tavistock, 1983

Cohen ML, Garofalo RF, Boucher R, et al: The psychology of rapists. Seminars in Psychiatry 3:307–327, 1971

Coid JW: DSM-III diagnosis in criminal psychopaths: a way forward. Criminal Behaviour and Mental Health 2:78–89, 1992

Coid JW: Current concepts and classifications of psychopathic disorder, in Personality Disorder Reviewed. Edited by Tyrer P, Stein G. London, Royal College of Psychiatrists, Gaskell, 1993a, pp 113–164

Coid JW: An affective syndrome in psychopaths with borderline personality disorder. Br J Psychiatry 162:641–650, 1993b

Coid J, Wilkins J, Coid B: Self-mutilation in female remanded prisoners II: a cluster analytic approach towards the identification of a behavioural syndrome. Criminal Behaviour and Mental Health 2:1–4, 1992

Crawford DA: The HDHQ results of long-term prisoners: relationships with criminal and institutional behaviour. Br J Clin Social Psychol 16:391–394, 1977

Digman JM: Personality structure: emergence of the five-factor model. Annu Rev Psychol 41:417–440, 1990

Dolan B, Coid J: Psychopathic and Antisocial Personality Disorders: Treatment and Research Issues. London, Royal College of Psychiatrists, Gaskell, 1993

Farrington DP: The development of offending and antisocial behaviour from childhood: key findings from the Cambridge study in delinquent development. J Child Psychol Psychiatry 360:929–964, 1995

Gebhard PH, Gagnon JH, Pomeroy WB, Christenson CV: Sex Offenders: An Analysis of Types. New York, Harper & Row, 1965

Gibbens TCN, Way C, Soothill KL: Behavioural types of rape. Br J Psychiatry 130:32–42, 1977

Groth AN, Birnbaum HJ: Men Who Rape: The Psychology of the Offender. New York, Plenum, 1979

Guttmacher MS: Sex Offenders: The Problem, Causes and Prevention. New York, WW Norton, 1951

Hare RD: The Hare Psychopathy Checklist—Revised Manual. Toronto, Multi-Health Systems, 1991

Henderson M: An empirical classification of convicted violent offenders. Br J Criminology 22:1–20, 1982

Henderson M: Self-reported assertion and aggression among violent offenders with high or low levels of overcontrolled hostility. Personality and Individual Differences 4:113–115, 1983

Henne RA, Herjanic M, Vanderpearl RH: Forensic psychiatry: profiles of two types of sex offender. Am J Psychiatry 133:694–696, 1976

Hesselbrock V, Stabenau J, Hesselbrock M, et al: A comparison of two interview schedules. Arch Gen Psychiatry 39:674–677, 1982

Hollin CR: Psychology and Crime. London, Routledge, 1989

Kernberg OF: Severe Personality Disorder. New Haven, CT, Yale University Press, 1984

Kohut H: Thoughts on narcissism and narcissistic rage. Psychoanal Study Child 27:360–400, 1973

Krakowski M, Volavka J, Brizer D: Psychopathology and violence: a review of the literature. Compr Psychiatry 27:131–148, 1986

Litwack TR, Schlesinger LB: Assessing and predicting violence: research, law and applications, in Handbook of Forensic Psychology. Edited by Weiner IB, Hess AK. New York, Wiley, 1987, pp 205–257

MacCulloch MJ, Snowden PR, Wood PJW, et al: Sadistic fantasy, sadistic behaviour and offending. Br J Psychiatry 143:20–29, 1983

McGurk BJ: Personality types among normal homicides. Br J Criminology 19:31–49, 1978

Mitchell B: Murder and Penal Policy. Basingstoke, Macmillan, 1990

Megargee EI: Undercontrolled and overcontrolled personality types in extreme antisocial aggression. Psychol Monogr 80(3):611, 1966

Monahan J, Klassen D: Situational approaches to understanding and predicting individual violent behaviour, in Criminal Violence. Edited by Wolfgang ME, Winer NA. Beverly Hills, CA, Sage, 1982

Prentsky R, Cohen M, Seghorn T: Development of a rational taxonomy for the classification of rapists: the Massachusetts treatment center system. Bull Am Acad Psychiatry Law 13:39–70, 1985

Quinsey VL, Maguire A, Varney GW: Assertion and overcontrolled hostility among mentally disordered murderers. J Consult Clin Psychol 51:550–556, 1983

Rada RT: Classification of the rapist, in Clinical Aspects of the Rapist. Edited by Rada RT. New York, Grune & Stratton, 1978

Raine A, Brenan P, Mendick SA: Birth complications combined with early maternal rejection at age 1 year predispose to violent crime at age 18 years. Arch Gen Psychiatry 51:984–988, 1994

Ressler RK, Burgess AW, Douglas JE: Sexual Homicide: Patterns and Motives. New York, Lexington Books, 1988

Ressler RK, Douglas JE, Burgess AW, et al: Crime Classification Manual. London, Simon & Schuster, 1993

Robins LN, Helzer JE, Croughan J, Ratcliff KS: National Institute of Health Diagnostic Interview Schedule—its history, characteristics and validity. Arch Gen Psychiatry 38:381–389, 1981

Rosen I: Perversion as a regulator of self-esteem, in Sexual Deviation, 2nd Edition. Edited by Rosen I. Oxford, Oxford University Press, 1979

Rosen I: Self-Esteem as a Factor in Social and Domestic Violence. Br J Psychiatry 158:18–23, 1991

Spitzer RL, Endicott J: Schedule for Affective Disorders and Schizophrenia—Lifetime Version, 3rd Edition. New York, New York State Psychiatric Institute, 1978

Spitzer RC, Williams E: Structural Clinical Interview for DSM-III Disorders (SCID). New York, New York State Psychiatric Institute, Biometric Research Department, 1983

Spitzer R, Endicott J, Robins E: Research Diagnostic Criteria for a Selected Group of Functional Disorders, 3rd Edition. New York, New York State Psychiatric Institute, 1978

Toch H, Adams K, Grant JG: Coping: Maladaption in Prisons. New Brunswick, NJ, Transaction Publishers, 1989

Widiger TA, Trull TJ: Personality disorders and violence, in Violence and Mental Disorder. Developments in Risk Assessment. Edited by Monahan J, Steadman HJ. Chicago, IL, University of Chicago Press, 1994, pp 203–226

Wing L: Asperger's syndrome: a clinical account. Psychol Med 11:115–129, 1983

Wolff S, Chick J: Schizoid personality in childhood: a controlled follow-up study. Psychol Med 10:85–100, 1980

Chapter 4

Biology of Aggression: Relevance to Crime

Emil F. Coccaro, M.D., and Brian McNamee, M.D., J.D.

Crime is the commission of any act that a lawful government deems illegal and punishable by incarceration and/or financial penalties. In the criminal justice system, criminal acts punishable by incarceration for 1 year or less are called misdemeanors; those punishable by incarceration for more than 1 year are called felonies.

Although the commission of a crime constitutes a behavioral act, the criminal act itself is not recognized as a psychiatric phenomenon. In DSM-IV (American Psychiatric Association 1994), simple acts of crime can only be coded under the V code of "adult antisocial behavior." However, if the acts of crime cluster with a variety of other behaviors and personality traits, and have been present before the age of 15, a diagnosis of antisocial personality disorder (ASPD) can be made. Barring this, a diagnosis of intermittent explosive disorder (IED) can be made if the acts of crime are violent and result in a serious assault against persons or in the destruction of property.

This brief review of the DSM reveals that psychiatry offers few options in the classification of criminal behavior. This is not surprising. Historically, criminal acts have not been thought to result from defective mental processes that fall within the rubric of psychiatric study and treatment. Instead, these acts have been thought of as volitional illegal acts unencumbered by aberrant mental or neurobiological processes. Even if these criminal acts occur in the context of an ASPD, the presence of personality disorder does not exculpate the perpetrator of the crime. This is because the presence of the personality disorder does not affect the ability of the individual's knowing the difference between right and wrong or the consequences of his or her act.

A more important problem for psychiatry in this regard is the concern that allowing a specific diganosis for criminal behavior will be used to excuse these behaviors, affecting jury verdicts and sentencing decisions. For example, if criminal behavior is inherently psychopathological, should criminals receive psychiatric treatment rather than incarceration? If so, what treatment? For the most part, psychiatric treatments for ASPD are ineffective, and there are no known treatments for IED.

Dealing with crime through standard psychiatric paradigms, however, is inherently unproductive. First, crime is not a unitary concept. There is violent and nonviolent crime and, among these, premeditated and nonpremeditated crime. Second, criminal acts occur in the context of a variety of developmental, social, and economic backgrounds. For example, a person who commits a crime given certain specific environmental conditions may not do so under different environmental conditions. Third, the interplay between temperament and character complicates the nature of crime, particularly as it relates to psychiatric study and treatment.

The last issue is extremely important and allows potentially for a paradigm shift in the study of selected criminal behavior in subsets of individuals. Temperament is a person's tendency to view and respond to his or her outer world in a specific and typical fashion. Temperament is dimensional and relatively specific (e.g., extraversion vs. introversion), significantly heritable, noticeable in very early life, and correlated with a variety of biological variables. Character, more complex by contrast, is the expression of a person's value system related to self and others (e.g., conscientiousness vs. nonconscientiousness). It is highly influenced by rearing environment and life experience, and less by genetic and biological factors. Accordingly, it is possible that biogenetic temperaments, rather than complex nonbiogenetic character styles, associated with criminal acts could be productive targets for biological study and treatment as they relate to criminal behavior. If certain predisposing temperaments are associated with abnormalities of neurobiological function, is it possible that correction of these abnormalities will reduce or eliminate the potential for criminal behavior?

Types of Criminal Behavior

A full review of the typology of criminal behavior is beyond the scope of this chapter. Accordingly, we will limit our discussion to only those issues relevant to the potential biological nature of criminal behavior.

The two most important phenomenological distinctions in criminal behavior from the biological point of view are the violent versus nonviolent and the impulsive versus nonimpulsive nature of criminal acts. Violent crime denotes criminal acts involving aggression against persons. These acts include homicide, attempted homicide, and other serious physical assault. Nonviolent crime usually refers to property crimes such as theft. The modifier impulsive/nonimpulsive refers to the issue of premeditation. Crimes not involving premediation are considered impulsive while crimes involving premeditation are considered nonimpulsive. In general, most data support the idea that impulsive violent criminal behavior has significant biological underpinnings that might lead to a rationale for pharmacological treatment. These data, as well as related data regarding impulsive aggression in noncriminal populations, are reviewed in greater detail in the following sections.

Genetic Studies of Crime and Aggression

Twin and Adoption Studies of Crime and Aggression

The hypothesis that crime, or aggression more generally, is influenced by genetic factors can be tested by a variety of methodologies. The most powerful of these include twin and adoption studies. In twin studies, the concordance for a particular condition among monozygotic twins is compared with that among dizygotic twins; in addition, heritability estimates can be calculated for continuous variables. Since monozygotic (MZ) twins share 100%, and dizygotic (DZ) twins only 50%, of their genetic endowment, a greater degree of concordance for a condition among MZ than among DZ twins suggests a genetic component (i.e., heritability) to the condition under study.

Twin studies of adult criminality have been limited in number. Christiansen (1968) reported a significant difference in concordance for criminality for MZ and DZ twins (74% vs. 47%) and suggested a substantial degree of heritability for criminal behavior. Other studies have also yielded differences of lower magnitude in MZ/DZ concordance that nevertheless suggested heritability. Dalgard and Kringlen (1976) reported a modest, but nonsignificant, difference in MZ/DZ concordance of 41% versus 26% using a definition of criminality that was confined to violent crime, sexual assault, theft, and robbery. Later, Christiansen (1977) reported a similar, though greater, difference in MZ/DZ concordance of 35% versus 13%. A recent twin study of self-reported criminality reported modest, but statistically significant, heritability estimates from .30 to .39 for arrests and/or criminal behavior occurring after the age of 15 (Lyons 1995). However, these twin studies generally treated criminality as a unitary variable. Accordingly, the issue of the heritability of violent crime, specifically, has not been formally addressed. An indirect answer to this question may be found in the twin study literature of aggressive behavior in which a small, but growing, number of studies in adult twins report significant heritabilities for a variety of self-report questionnaire measures of aggression (Miles and Carey 1997). Differentiating between types of aggression, we have recently reported that direct physical aggression demonstrates the greatest heritability: 47% heritability for direct physical aggression versus 40% for indirect physical aggression versus 28% for verbal aggression (Coccaro et al. 1997a).

Although twin studies can establish whether a genetic influence on a condition exists, the assessment of environmental influences is more difficult. Before the establishment of twin cohorts reared apart and together and the development of sophisticated statistical modeling procedures, the only method available to assess genetic and environmental issues simultaneously was the adoption study method. In adoption studies, the frequency of the condition under study in individuals adopted away from their biological parents with and without the condition is assessed. Accordingly, four types of cells are constructed in this design: 1) children of affected parents reared by nonaffected adoptive parents; 2) children of affected parents reared by affected adoptive parents; 3) children of nonaffected parents reared by affected adoptive parents; and 4) children of nonaffected parents reared by nonaffected adoptive parents. This methodology allows estimates of the effects of both genetic and environmental influences as well as of gene-environment interactions on the condition in question.

One of the first adoption studies of criminality, reported by Hutchings and Mednick (1973), examined 14,427 nonfamilial adoptions in Denmark from 1924 to 1947. In this study, a significant relationship was found between the number of convictions among the biological parents, particularly fathers, and the rate of convictions among the adopted-away sons. A similar relationship was seen when chronic offending in the parents was examined separately. Surprisingly, only property offending in adoptees was related to criminal offending in biological parents; violent offending in adoptees did not correlate with violent offending in the biological parents.

These data are generally consistent with those of other investigators. In an American study, Crowe (1974) reported 7 criminal offenders among the 52 adopted-away offspring of incarcerated women, compared with only 1 offender in the matched control group. In a later study, Bohman et al. (1982) discovered that petty, but not violent, criminality was heritable if child and biological parent did not meet criteria for alcohol abuse. If child or biological parent had both criminality and alcohol abuse, the criminality was usually symptomatic of the alcoholism. When Bohman (1978) reexamined his previously negative results, he found an excess of criminality alone in sons of biological fathers with criminality alone. In a subsequent analysis of these data, Cloninger et al. (1982) reported that 59% of the variability in petty criminality in the sample could be explained by genetic influence, 19% by environmental influence, 14% by gene-environment interaction, and 7% by gene-environment correlation. In general, low social status did not increase the risk for petty criminality unless the father of the adoptee was a criminal or if the mother of the adoptee was an alcoholic.

Given that aggressive behavior is moderately heritable (Miles and Carey 1997), data suggesting that violent criminality may not be heritable are curious. It is possible that violent behavior in the adoptees of previous studies results from an interaction between criminality and psychiatric disorder (e.g., schizophrenia) in the biological parent (Brennan et al. 1996). It is also possible that it is difficult to detect a heritability signal for violent criminality because it is far less frequent than property/petty criminality and because violent offenders commit a significant number of property/petty offenses as well.

Chromosomal Abnormalities

Although the genetic influences underlying criminal and/or aggressive behavior must reside in the genetic code contained within the genome, early efforts to physically relate these behaviors to the genome focused on testing for chromosomal abnormalities. The most widely studied chromosomal abnormalities in this regard were the XYY and XXY karyotypes. The earliest studies reported a higher than expected frequency of criminality among mental hospital patients with either karyotype (Neilson 1970). A later study also found a higher than expected frequency of these karyotypes in a criminal population (Neilson and Hendrikson 1972). These data were supported by findings from other studies (Hamerton 1976; Murken 1973; Nanko et al. 1979; Noel and Benezech 1977; Witken et al. 1976). The mechanism of this association is not known; however, many XYY males have been reported to have diminished intelligence and poor emotional control (Hunter 1977), factors that increase the risk of criminal behavior. In addition, both XYY and XXY males have been shown to demonstrate slow alpha frequency on EEG evaluation (Frey 1975). This feature suggests that the presence of an additional sex chromosome, be it an X or a Y, is associated with a developmental defect in the central nervous system, which in turn increases the risk of deviant, if not criminal, behavior. However, despite the statistical association between these karyotypes and criminality, it should be emphasized that XYY or XXY individuals compose a very small proportion of the criminal population and, compared with normal males, manifest only minor differences in aggression (Schiavi et al. 1984).

DNA Polymorphisms

More informative than karyotyping, the study of DNA polymorphisms is currently being applied to the study of psychiatric disorders. DNA polymorphisms represent variants in DNA sequences within genes. These variants may be in coding (exons) or noncoding regions (introns) of the gene. If the variant is in a coding region, it is possible that one form (allele) of the gene may represent a mutation and lead to, for example, less gene product (protein) than is necessary for neuronal function. If the variant is in a noncoding region, the polymorphism may have either no functional significance or be in linkage with an unknown polymorphism that affects a functional gene product.

To date, the best-characterized DNA polymorphism related to criminality or aggression is a polymorphism within the tryptophan hydroxylase (TPH) gene. TPH is the rate-limiting enzyme in the synthesis of serotonin (5-hydroxytryptamine [5-HT]), a neurotransmitter long associated with impulsive aggressive behavior in humans (see following). Recently, Nielson et al. (1994) reported that impulsive violent offenders with one or two copies of the TPH "L" allele had significantly lower cerebrospinal fluid (CSF) concentrations of 5-hydroxyindoleacetic acid (5-HIAA), the major CSF metabolite for 5-HT, than impulsive violent offenders with two copies of the "U" allele. Curiously, this relationship was not observed among nonimpulsive violent offenders or among normal controls, suggesting a complex relationship between TPH allelic status, CSF 5-HIAA, and impulsive criminality. Although TPH allelic status did not distinguish impulsive from nonimpulsive violent offenders, the presence an an "L" allele in either group was associated with a greater proportion with a life history of a suicide attempt (LL: 65% vs. LU: 53% vs. UU: 17%, $P < .02$). The presence of an "LL" genotype has also been shown to be associated with self-reported aggressive tendencies in a group of Caucasian males with personality disorder (New et al., in press). A study conducted in the laboratory of one of the authors using a life history measure of actual aggressive events in similarly defined individuals with personality disorder does not replicate this finding (E. Coccaro, unpublished data, September 1997). However, the fact that this polymorphism is not in the coding region of the TPH gene may account for differences in findings among study samples. It is possible, for example, that the TPH polymorphism may be in linkage dysequilibrium with a relevant but unknown polymorphism in one study sample and not in the other.

Biological Studies of Crime and Aggression

Neurotransmitter Mediators in the Study of Crime and Aggression

Serotonin. Evidence suggesting a role of central 5-HT in impulsive aggression in humans is strong. Inverse correlations between CSF 5-HIAA concentrations and life history of actual aggressive events (Brown et al. 1979) and of self-reported deviant (Brown et al. 1982) and aggressive (Brown and Goodwin 1984) tendencies in adult males were first reported in the late 1970s and early 1980s. The idea that reduced central 5-HT function was more specifically associated with impulsive aggression was first advanced by Linnoila et al. (1983), who showed that CSF 5-HIAA concentrations among impulsive violent offenders were lower than those among nonimpulsive violent offenders. Among all violent offenders, individuals with a history of repeated violent offenses had lower CSF 5-HIAA concentrations than those who had committed only one violent offense. Later, Virkkunen et al. (1987) showed that arsonists who were impulsive, but not necessarily interpersonally violent, also had reduced CSF 5-HIAA concentrations in comparison to normal controls. Although these data suggest a primacy for impulsivity over aggression with regard to central 5-HT function, evidence from later studies (see following) suggest that the critical phenomenologic factor may be impulsive aggression rather than impulsivity alone.

A number of other, though not all, CSF 5-HIAA studies in human and nonhuman primates support the role of central 5-HT in impulsive aggression, if not impulsivity itself. Inverse correlations between CSF 5-HIAA and measures of aggression have been reported in abstinent alcoholic individuals (Limson et al. 1991), in children and adolescents with disruptive behavior disorders (Kruesi et al. 1990), and in rhesus monkeys (Higley et al. 1992; Mehlman et al. 1994). Moreover, the finding that impulsive violent offenders have lower CSF 5-HIAA concentrations than nonimpulsive violent offenders has been replicated (Virkkunen et al. 1994). In addition, CSF 5-HIAA concentrations have been reported as low in recidivistic violent offenders (Virkkunen et al. 1989a) and in violent offenders with a personal history of suicide attempt (Linnoila et al. 1983; Virkkunen et al. 1989b) or with a history of paternal alcoholism (Linnoila et al. 1989).

In contrast to these data, at least five studies regarding CSF 5-HIAA do not report an inverse correlation with measures of aggression. Three report no such correlation in participants with personality disorder (Gardner et al. 1990; Coccaro 1992; Coccaro et al. 1997b), and two report a positive correlation in participants with attention-deficit/hyperactivity disorder (Castellanos et al. 1994) or in normal persons (Moller et al. 1996). Careful review of these studies suggests that the severity of aggressive behavior probably accounts for the differences among studies reporting, and not reporting, inverse relationships between CSF 5-HIAA concentration and aggression. Aggressive behavior in positive reports was often characterized as very severe and resulted in criminal (Linnoila et al. 1983; Virkkunen et al. 1994) or military judicial (Brown et al. 1979, 1982) penalties. Although the aggressive behavior of participants in the negative reports was clinically significant, it did not reach this level of severity. Given this differential in the "severity of aggression," it is possible that there would be no inverse relationship with aggression despite which index of central 5-HT function was used. However, evidence of an inverse relationship with central 5-HT and aggression was noted in two of the studies (Coccaro 1992; Coccaro et al. 1997b) when a physiologic index of 5-HT (i.e., hormonal response to 5-HT stimulation) was used. This suggests that although CSF 5-HIAA measures often correlate inversely with aggression in severely aggressive individuals, such measures might not correlate inversely in less severely aggressive participants; in the latter group, a physiologic assessment of 5-HT responsiveness may be more sensitive.

Other methods for assessing central 5-HT system function have also demonstrated inverse relationships between 5-HT and impulsive aggression. The two most frequently used methods in this regard involve: 1) hormonal responses to acute pharmacological stimulation of central 5-HT synapses, and 2) measurement of platelet 5-HT receptors. In the first method, an acute dose of a 5-HT pharmacologic agent is given, and the peripheral hormonal response is measured over time. Because this response is dose related and begins in the limbic hypothalamus, the magnitude of the hormonal response to pharmacologic challenge is taken as an index of the scalar responsivity of the 5-HT synapses in the limbic hypothalamus (Coccaro and Kavoussi 1994). In the second method, the number of 5-HT transporter and 5-HT$_{2A}$ receptor binding sites are measured. Since the neuronal and platelet receptors for these two sites are nearly identical from a molecular standpoint (Cook et al. 1994; Lesch et al. 1993), platelet 5-HT receptors are taken as models of the same receptors on central neurons.

Pharmacological challenge studies of aggressive individuals were first published in the late 1980s. The first comprehensive study utilizing this methodology, conducted with patients with personality disorder (Coccaro et al. 1989), reported an inverse relationship between the prolactin response to d,l-fenfluramine (PRL[d,l-FEN]) and measures of aggression (i.e., life history of aggression, self-reported assault, and irritability) and impulsivity. When each of these measures was examined in the same regression model, aggression, but not impulsivity, remained associated with reduced PRL[d,l-FEN] responses in these patients. Although impulsivity correlated highly with the aggression variables, impulsivity did not uniquely contribute to the model above and beyond that contributed by aggression variables. Other important relationships were noted as well. These included an inverse relationship between PRL[d,l-FEN] and current diagnosis of borderline personality disorder, past history of suicide attempt, and past history of alcoholism. Each of these factors correlated directly with the aggression variables, however, and when each was examined in the same regression model, only the aggression variables contributed uniquely to the model. Accordingly, these data suggested that the strongest behavioral correlate of reduced PRL[d,l-FEN] responses, as an index of central 5-HT system function, was the type of aggression that had shared variance with impulsivity (i.e., "impulsive aggression").

These findings were generally confirmed in many, though not all, subsequent studies. In participants with personality disorder, inverse relationships have been reported between aggression variables and PRL responses to d,l-FEN (New et al. 1997; Siever and Trestman 1993; Stein et al. 1996), d-FEN (Coccaro et al. 1996a, 1997b), the 5-HT$_{1A}$ probes buspirone (Coccaro et al. 1990) and ipsapirone (Coccaro et al. 1995), and the 5-HT$_{1A/2C}$ probe m-chlorophenylpiperazine (m-CPP) (Moss et al. 1990). In violent offenders, PRL[d-FEN] responses have been reported to be reduced compared with normal controls (O'Keane et al. 1992). In nonhuman primates, reduced PRL[d,l-FEN] responses are associated with high ratings of overt aggression (Botchin et al. 1993). In alcoholic participants, PRL[m-CPP] responses have been reported to correlate inversely with self-reported aggressive tendencies (Handelsman et al. 1996). Negative studies in this area have also been published. In adult participants, these include studies of individuals with mood disorder (Coccaro et al. 1989; Wetzler et al. 1991) or anxiety disorder (Wetzler et al. 1991). In general drug-abusing (Fishbein et al. 1989) and cocaine-abusing (Bernstein and Handelsman 1995) participants, positive relationships between PRL responses to d,l-FEN and m-CPP, respectively, and self-reported aggressive and impulsive tendencies have been reported. In these cases, it is possible that the presence of certain (e.g., mood or anxiety) disorders or the pharmacologic effect of a long history of illicit (nonalcohol) drug use alters the biological substrate of the participants so that an inverse relationship between 5-HT and aggression is not observed or is reversed. In children and adolescents, PRL[d,l-FEN] responses have been reported to be positively related to aggression (Halperin et al. 1994; Pine et al. 1997) or not related to aggression at all (Halperin et al. 1997; Stoff et al. 1992). These differences may be due to age and developmental factors. In both studies where a positive relationship between PRL[d,l-FEN] responses and aggression was seen, the participants were younger than those individuals in studies where no relationship was seen. It is possible that differential development of the central 5-HT system may occur in aggressive children (Halperin et al. 1997). According to this model, aggressive children may demonstrate a positive relationship between 5-HT and aggression, which becomes null during adolescence, then inverse in nature as adulthood is reached.

Studies involving platelet 5-HT measures were also first published in the late 1980s. Stoff et al. (1987) reported that aggressive children with conduct disorder had lower numbers of ^{3}H-imipramine binding sites on platelets than did nonaggressive children with conduct disorder. Although Stoff's group could not replicate this finding, another group reported a similar result (Birmaher et al. 1990). In addition, other investigators reported similar findings in studies of persons with mental retardation or of other institutionalized persons (Marazziti et al. 1993). Most recently, Coccaro et al. (1996b) reported an inverse correlation between the numbers of platelet ^{3}H-paroxetine binding sites and life history of actual aggressive events. Coccaro's group also reported a positive relationship between the number of 5-HT$_{2A}$ receptor binding sites, reduced receptor affinity, and self-reported aggressive tendencies (Coccaro et al. 1997c).

Norepinephrine and dopamine.   Animal studies suggest a facilitory role for both norepinephrine and dopamine with regard to aggression (Coccaro 1996), but supporting data from clinical studies are limited. Brown et al. (1979) reported a positive correlation between the CSF concentration of norepinephrine's major metabolite, 3-methoxy-4-hydroxyphenylglycol (MHPG), and life history of aggressive events in 12 men with personality disorder. However, when both CSF 5-HIAA and MHPG concentrations were examined in the same statistical model, CSF 5-HIAA accounted for 80% of the variance in aggression. In contrast to this, Virkkunen et al. (1987) reported significantly lower CSF MHPG in violent offenders and in impulsive arsonists compared with healthy volunteers. In subsequent studies, however, CSF MHPG was not found to differ as a function of violent offending or recidivism (Virkkunen et al. 1989a, 1994).

Clinical evidence for a role of dopamine in aggression and/or criminality is similarly limited. Reduced CSF concentrations of homovanillic acid (HVA), the major dopamine metabolite, was initially reported among impulsive violent offenders with antisocial personality (but not IED only) by Linnoila et al. (1983). Although this finding was not replicated in later studies by Virkkunen et al. (1987, 1994), reduced CSF HVA concentration has been reported as a function of recidivism in the offender (Virkkunen et al. 1989a) and as a function of violent behavior in the offender's father (Virkkunen et al. 1996). Inverse relationships between CSF HVA and aggression have also been reported in abstinent alcoholic persons and healthy volunteers (Limson et al. 1991). Interpretation of these findings is complicated by the fact that CSF 5-HIAA and HVA are highly intercorrelated, and CSF HVA may be "driven" by CSF 5-HIAA (Agren et al. 1986). Accordingly, it is possible that CSF HVA findings merely reflect the primary finding with CSF 5-HIAA concentration. Unfortunately, none of the published studies previously cited examined the relationship between CSF HVA and criminality/aggression in the context of its relationship with CSF 5-HIAA. In our laboratory we have found that CSF HVA can correlate inversely with life history measures of aggressive events in individuals with personality disorder even after the effect of CSF 5-HIAA is accounted for. If this is true for violent offender populations, CSF HVA may have important scientific value in this regard.

Vasopressin. Animal studies suggest a facilitory role for central vasopressin in aggressive behavior. In the golden hamster, for example, administration of vasopressin receptor antagonists reduces aggressive behavior (Ferris and Delville 1994). In the same animal model, enhancement of 5-HT activity by fluoxetine had been shown to reduce aggression and to reduce central vasopressin levels, suggesting that vasopressin may work in concert with 5-HT to modulate aggressive behavior (Delville et al. 1996). Recently, we reported that CSF vasopressin correlates directly with life history measures of aggression in individuals with personality disorder (Coccaro et al. 1996c). Although PRL[d-FEN] responses were inversely correlated with aggression, and with CSF vasopressin, in the same participants the direct relationship with CSF vasopressin remained even after accounting for the relationship with the 5-HT index, PRL[d-FEN] response.

Metabolic and Hormonal Mediators in the Study of Crime and Aggression

Glucose metabolism.   In the 1970s sporadic reports were published suggesting an association between hypoglycemia and aggression (Bovill 1973; Groesbeck et al. 1975; Yarura-Tobias and Neziroglu 1975). Glucose is the primary energy source in the brain. Accordingly, significant hypoglycemia is thought to lead to impaired central neuronal function and consequent impairment in cognitive processes and judgment (O'Keefe and Marks 1977), which can increase the risk for aggressive responding in the context of aversive external stimuli.

Systematic follow-up investigation of this work by Virkkunen has documented a clear link between reactive hypoglycemia and history of impulsive aggression, specifically in violent offenders who committed their violent acts under the influence of alcohol. In a series of investigations, Virkkunen and colleagues demonstrated that both impulsive violent offenders with ASPD (Virkkunen and Huttunen 1982), or with IED (Virkkunen 1982, 1984; Virkkunen et al. 1994), had a significantly lower glucose nadir after glucose challenge compared with normal volunteers. Since most of the violent offenders had committed their crimes under the influence of alcohol, itself associated with an enhanced insulinemic and hypoglycemic response to glucose challenge (Nikkila and Taskinen 1975), it is likely that neuroglycopenia contributed to the conditions under which their violent behavior occurred.

Subgroup analysis involving these participants proved revealing. For example, impulsive violent offenders with criminal fathers had lower glucose nadirs than those without criminal fathers (Virkkunen 1982), suggesting a familial/genetic component to the reactive hypoglycemia manifested by these participants. Curiously, antisocial violent offenders had a longer period of reactive hypoglycemia than those with IED, suggesting a potential difference between the two that may relate to the possibility that persons with ASPD might have a widepread abnormality in various homeostatic mechanisms (Mawson and Mawson 1977). Further study confirmed that impulsive violent offenders with ASPD had an elevated insulin response to glucose challenge that was not present in similar individuals with ASPD who were not particularly aggressive (Virkkunen 1983a). Among violent offenders, the hypoglycemic response to glucose challenge has also been found to be greater among recidivists who have committed new violent crimes (Virkkunen et al. 1989a). Notably, the blood glucose nadir value correctly classified recidivists 80.7% of the time.

Since reactive hypoglycemia and low CSF 5-HIAA concentration may both be characteristic of impulsive violent offenders, it is reasonable to hypothesize that these variables are linked in some way. However, unlike CSF 5-HIAA concentrations (see earlier), no differences in blood glucose nadir have been found for the factors of history of suicide attempt (Virkkunen et al. 1989b) or presence of an alcoholic father (Linnoila et al. 1989) in violent offenders. Accordingly, reactive hypoglycemia and low CSF 5-HIAA concentration may represent different risk factors for violence in violent offenders.

Testosterone.   Although the facilitory role of testosterone in aggressive behavior is well documented in animal studies, support for this role in humans is less clear (Archer 1991). This is related to a variety of factors, including the form of testosterone measured (free vs. bound), the bodily fluid compartment studied (plasma vs. saliva vs. CSF), choice of behavioral variables (aggression vs. hostility vs. competitiveness), and the type of individual studied (normal volunteers vs. athletes vs. clinical participants). In general, there appears to be a modest positive relationship between testosterone and competitiveness and aggression/hostility when free testosterone is measured in plasma or saliva in normal volunteers or athletes. In clinical participants, particularly impulsive violent offenders, CSF free testosterone has been reported to be elevated in antisocial, but not intermittently explosive, individuals (Virkkunen et al. 1994). It is unknown why the latter subgroup of impulsive violent offenders do not show elevated CSF free testosterone.

Cortisol and corticotropin. The role of cortisol and corticotropin in violence has had limited study to date, with most of this work reported by Virkkunen and collegues. In 1985 Virkkunen reported that 24-hour urinary free cortisol was low in antisocial, but not in intermittently explosive or nonimpulsive, violent offenders. In another study (Virkkunen et al. 1994), CSF corticotropin was reported to be significantly reduced in antisocial impulsive violent offenders compared with healthy volunteers. However, while only this comparison was reported as statistically significant, the means for the intermittently explosive violent offenders and the nonimpulsive violent offenders were only slightly higher than that for the antisocial impulsive violent offenders. Reasons for nonsignificance in the comparison with the healthy volunteers include the small sample sizes ($n = 13$ to 17 per cell) and the lower variablity in CSF corticotropin levels among the antisocial impulsive violent offenders.

One possible mechanism for a role of cortisol in aggression relates to its effect on increasing the affinity of central testosterone receptors. In animal studies, adrenalectomized rats have been reported to 1) develop spontaneous aggressive behavior within 24 hours of surgery and 2) require only low doses of exogenous testosterone to elicit sustained attack behavior (Essman 1981). A possible role for corticotropin in aggression, aside from its effect on circulating cortisol levels, is unknown.

Cholesterol. A potential relationship between serum cholesterol and violence has been reported since the late 1970s. Virkkunen (1979) first reported a low serum cholesterol level among antisocial, compared with other, non-antisocial, participants with personality disorder. Nearly all the antisocial participants had committed property crimes, but only slightly more than half had committed a violent offense. However, in a second study involving a large group of homicide offenders, Virkkunen (1983b) demonstrated that impulsive violent offenders (either with ASPD or IED) also had lower serum cholesterol levels than nonimpulsive violent offenders. Among all homicide offenders, the presence of a personal history of suicide attempt, self-injurious behavior, and the presence of paternal violence under the influence of alcohol were all associated with lower serum cholesterol levels.

Given this pattern of findings, similar to that seen with indices of 5-HT (see earlier), it is possible that serum cholesterol bears some relationship with central 5-HT function. Recent studies performed in the monkey suggest this may be true (Kaplan et al. 1994). In these studies, monkeys were fed low- and high-cholesterol diets to produce hypocholesterolemic and hypercholesterolemic monkeys, respectively. As predicted, hypocholesterolemic monkeys were more aggressive than hypercholesterolemic monkeys. In addition, hypocholesterolemic monkeys had lower CSF 5-HIAA concentrations than did hypercholesterolemic monkeys, supporting the hypothesis that serum cholesterol, at least in the extreme conditions employed in this study, is directly related to central 5-HT system function. Whether these relationships hold in humans, when only modest intraindividual differences in serum cholesterol are observed, is less clear. Although one study suggests a positive relationship between PRL[m-CPP] responses (Terao et al. 1997), another was unable to detect a reduction in PRL[d-FEN] responses in human participants treated with lipid-lowering agents (Delva et al. 1996).

A Case Study of Criminal Impulsive Violence

BC presented for a psychiatric evaluation as part of a criminal defense plea of not guilty by reason of insanity. At that time, BC was a 30-year-old, divorced, white male who was incarcerated awaiting his trial for the murder of his ex-wife. Until his incarceration for this crime, BC worked as an accountant at a small firm in a bedroom community of a major city. He had two young daughters by his ex-wife.

Personal history. BC was the oldest of four children. His mother noted early problems with impulsive behavior and anger control. She noted that as a child, BC was particularly apt to react with rage when he felt that he had been wronged by someone. He was hyperactive, likely to wander off away from home or run away from home if he felt he had been unfairly treated. His early school years were noteworthy for hyperactivity and fighting, as well as fire setting, by the age of 6 to 7 years. Evidence of his impulsive aggressive behavior included an incident in which he intentionally, reactively severed the tip of his 3-year-old brother's fifth finger during an altercation, when he himself was 5 years old. By the second grade, BC described himself as a "runt with a mouth." He attended a private school from grades 1 through 6 but was asked to leave that school because of an inability to control his rage. At the age of 7, in the second grade, he assaulted his teacher because she had "smacked him" for noisy misbehavior. By the sixth grade, he had struck another teacher for a "forgotten minor reason." This resulted in a visit to the principal's office, further enragement, and a verbal threat to "shoot" the teacher. This threat resulted in his expulsion. During this period, BC engaged in aggressive behaviors that generally involved fighting with other children when he felt he had been unfairly treated; there was, however, no history to suggest that he behaved as a "bully" in the sense of taking advantage of younger or smaller children. Despite these behaviors, his academic performance was always high, grades ranging from As to Bs, with evidence of perfectionist and obsessive tendencies in his schoolwork.

Entering high school, BC continued to engage in episodic fighting but, by all accounts, only when challenged. His academic performance continued to be high, with a good grade point average. Upon finishing high school at the age of 17 years, he had a physical fight with his father and left home, then joined the army. He was honorably discharged 4 years later but recounts a number of violent incidents during his time in the army. He received high praise and rapid promotions in the army for excellent organizational skills, timely and creative completion of tasks, and reliability. There were, however, at least two incidents of alleged assaults, one in a barroom brawl and a second for striking a sergeant who he felt had treated him unfairly.

During his college years, BC apparently began to exhibit identifiable fluctuations in mood. College roommates reported that he would go for long periods apparently requiring little sleep. He carried a full college load, with a triple major, and worked in the evenings. He seemed to be able to study and do his schoolwork until early hours of the morning, arise after only a few hours of sleep, and attend classes the next day. Alternately, however, he appeared to enter periods during which he would isolate himself from others, stay in his room, and not communicate. During this time BC worked regularly, occasionally as a barroom bouncer. BC estimates that he had more than 100 physical fights in his lifetime and had been arrested for fighting on at least 12 occasions.

BC met his ex-wife, a salesclerk, in the interval between his discharge from the army and his enrollment in college. BC maintained intermittent contact with this woman, and they were eventually married during BC's second year of school, when she became pregnant. The ex-wife's past history is noteworthy for a history of substance abuse, including marijuana and cocaine abuse, impulsivity, and violent behavior.

A second child was born to the couple during BC's third year at college. However, trouble in the marriage led the couple to maintain separate residences. Shortly after BC's graduation from college, his wife informed him that she desired a divorce. Following divorce, serious problems arose over child visitation issues. After numerous disputes with his ex-wife, the most recent of which led to BC's violation of a restraining order, BC obtained a 9-millimeter semiautomatic handgun and started drinking more than ususal. BC developed a plan to kill himself in front of his ex-wife. He felt that he was going to go to jail for violating her restraining order for a second time. As a consequence, he reasoned that his wife would obtain full custody of the children. Since she had "beaten him," he decided he would kill himself in front of her, leaving splattered brains on her kitchen wall for her to explain to his children. When BC arrived at his ex-wife's house, she ran from the house and went to her neighbor. As his initial plan went awry, BC instantly became enraged. He followed her to the next house, grabbed her, and killed her with a single shot to the head. Following 3 weeks of eluding the law enforcement authorities, during which time he continued to drink heavily, BC voluntarily presented himself to the local police authorities for prosecution.

Family history. Family history is remarkable for impulsive aggression, depression, and alcohol/substance abuse on both the paternal and maternal sides of BC's family. Among the 20 first- and second-degree family members for which information was available, 7 had had problems with impulsive aggression, 5 had had problems with alcohol/substance abuse, and 4 had had problems with depression.

Laboratory results. Although BC's CSF 5-HIAA level of 92.8 nmol/L was in the normal range of values reported in the literature, BC's CSF HVA level of 107 nmol/L would be considered low compared with healthy volunteers (Virkkunen et al. 1994). In addition, BC had a reduced PRL[d,l-FEN] response of 4.15 ng/ml (Coccaro et al. 1989). BC's hypoglycemic response of 51 mg/dl at 3 hours into the glucose tolerance test (GTT) was nearly abnormal (<50 mg/dl).

Discussion. BC is illustrative of the type of impulsive violent offender that has been studied and reported on in the biological psychiatry literature. First, BC meets criteria for IED. Impulsive violent offenders usually meet criteria for either IED or antisocial/borderline personality disorder. Second, his act of violence was impulsive in that he committed murder in an impulsive, reactive act of rage after his original plan was "ruined" by his ex-wife's actions (reportedly his plan was to commit suicide, not homicide). Although BC's act does not meet a legal definition of non-premediatation (i.e., where there is no conscious thought to kill before the act occurs), there was actually little premeditation or planning in the murder of his ex-wife. BC consciously, but impulsively, altered his plan from suicide to homicide at the scene of the crime. Third, his homicide was committed while under the influence of alcohol. (Note that though BC has been impulsively aggressive in the absence of alcohol, his more severe aggressive acts have occurred in the context of alcohol consumption.) Fourth, he has a childhood history of "hyperactivity." Fifth, he has a strong family history of impulsive aggressiveness and of alcoholism, particularly on the paternal side of his family.

BC's biological data is generally consistent with that reported in the literature. First, he has a reduced PRL[d,l-FEN] response. This suggests that when BC's central 5-HT neurons were stimulated to release 5-HT, the functional response was low compared with what is expected in normal males (Coccaro et al. 1989). Given a normal CSF 5-HIAA level (suggesting the presence of a normal number of functional 5-HT neurons presynaptically), these data suggest that the postsynaptic 5-HT receptors underlying BC's PRL[d,l-FEN] response are relatively insensitive to 5-HT stimulation. Second, he has a reduced CSF HVA level. Although not as consistent a finding as that with the CSF 5-HIAA level, CSF HVA levels have been shown to correlate inversely with measures of aggression (Limson et al. 1991), criminal recidivism (Virkkunen et al. 1989a), and paternal violence (Virkkunen et al. 1996). BC's reactive hypoglycemic response in the GTT is also consistent with what has been reported in impulsive violent offenders (Virkkunen 1982, 1984; Virkkunen et al. 1994). In the context of the specific crime, it is noteworthy that BC was drinking (and eating little) just prior to the crime. Given his propensity toward reactive hypoglycemia on the GTT, it is likely that BC was probably hypoglycemic and neuroglycopenic at the time of the crime. Since glucose is the primary energy source in the brain, neuroglycopenia could have significantly contributed to the impairment in cognitive processes and judgment (O'Keefe and Marks 1977) that BC appeared to have at the time of the crime.

The presence of these biological abnormalities in BC certainly does not excuse the fact that BC committed a homicide. Rather, it gives insight into the physiological risk factors that may underlie serious violent behavior, particularly if it is relatively impulsive in nature.

In the state in which BC's trial took place (and many other states), a defendant is not guilty by reason of insanity if, as a result of a "defect" or "disease" of the mind, he or she did not know the "wrongfulness" of his or her act. Accordingly, the defense must prove these two elements by a "preponderance of the evidence." In BC's case, the defense attempted to establish the first prong of the insanity defense by introducing evidence that BC was afflicted with an impulse control disorder, IED. Testimony was introduced summarizing his clinical history, which established that he fulfilled DSM-IV criteria for IED. Testimony was also introduced that BC suffered from an untreated form of bipolar disorder. It was the defense's contention that underlying these clinical disorders, particularly IED, was evidence of neurochemical abnormalities affecting both serotonin and dopamine pathways, as described earlier. In the time leading up to the killing, the defense also argued that BC was in a state of dysphoric mania (or hypomania), which would have increased the risk of an impulsive aggressive outburst typical of BC during his lifetime. This assertion regarding his mood state was corroborated by the testimony of numerous witnesses, including his girlfriend, who described profound symptoms of agitated depression and, at the same time, hypersexuality, just prior to and on the day of the homicide.

In addition, the defense was required to demonstrate that BC did not know the "wrongfulness" of his acts at the time he committed them. The presence of an "irresistible impulse," as suggested earlier, does not satisfy this criterion in the state of BC's trial (nor in most states). The defense's argument was that BC did not intend to kill his ex-wife in the immediate time period preceding the homicide. When his confused planning went awry,

BC responded impulsively and aggressively without reflection. Thus, the defense argued that BC was incapable of moral reflection in his unihibited rage state.

Regardless, the court was not persuaded that BC was not guilty by reason of insanity. BC was found guilty of murder in the first degree. Although the potentially mitigating clinical and biological data were available to the court during the penalty phase of BC's trial, the court rendered a sentence of death.

Conclusion

It is possible that our growing biological understanding of impulsive aggression will lead to a reconceptualization regarding the process of jury verdicts and sentencing in the case of impulsive violent crime. Pending further study and consideration, it is possible that some form of appropriate pharmacological treatment may be offered to selected impulsive violent offenders in addition to incarceration and currently available rehabilitation. For example, current pharmacological data suggest that some agents, such as lithium (Sheard et al. 1976) and anticonvulsants (Barratt et al. 1997), can reduce impulsive aggressiveness in criminal offenders. If so, violence risk, and prison terms, might be significantly reduced in selected individuals. Of course, much more research will be necessary in the relevant populations before this course of action could be applied in our criminal justice system. Review of the legal literature reveals that courts are extremely cautious regarding the role psychiatric evaluation and treatment plays in sentencing considerations and that the courts will require a very high standard of scientific proof before our current biological understanding of the impulsive violent offender has any impact on the judicial process (Denno 1996).

References

Agren H, Mefford IN, Rudorfer MV, et al: Interacting neurotransmitter systems: a non-experimental approach to the 5-HIAA-HVA correlation in human CSF. J Psychiatr Res 20:175–193, 1986

American Psychiatric Association: Diagnostic and Statistical Manual: Mental Disorders, 4th Edition. Washington, DC, American Psychiatric Association, 1994

Archer J: The influence of testosterone on human aggression. Br J Psychology 82:1–28, 1991

Barratt ES, Stanford MS, Felthous AR, et al: The effects of phenytoin on impulsive and premeditated aggression: a controlled study. J Clin Psychopharmacol 17:341–349, 1997

Bernstein DP, Handelsman L: The neurobiology of substance abuse and personality disorders, in Neuropsychiatry of Personality Disorders. Edited by Ratey JJ. Cambridge, MA, Blackwell Science, Inc., 1995, pp 120–148

Birmaher B, Stanley M, Greenhill L, et al: Platelet imipramine binding in children and adolescents with impulsive behavior. J Am Acad Child Adolesc Psychiatry 29:914–918, 1990

Bohman M: Some genetic aspects of alcoholism and criminality: a population of adoptees. Arch Gen Psychiatry 35:269–276, 1978

Bohman M, Cloninger RC, Sigvardsson S, et al: Predisposition to petty criminality in Swedish adoptees, I: genetic and environmental heterogeneity. Arch Gen Psychiatry 39:1233–1241, 1982

Botchin MB, Kaplan JR, Manuck SB, et al: Low versus high prolactin responders to fenfluramine challenge: marker of behavioral differences in adult male cynmolgus macaques. Neuropsychopharmacology 9:93–99, 1993

Bovill D: A case of functional hypoglycemia—a medicolegal problem. Br J Psychiatry 123:353–358, 1973

Brennan PA, Mednick SA, Jacobesen B: Assessing the role of genetics in crime using adoption cohorts, in Genetics of Criminal and Antisocial Behavior (Ciba Foundation Symposium). Chichester, Wiley, 1996, pp 115–128

Brown GL, Goodwin FK: Diagnostic, clinical and personality characteristics of aggressive men with low CSF 5-HIAA. Clin Neuropharmacol 7:S408-S409, 1984

Brown GL, Goodwin FK, Ballenger JC, et al: Aggression in humans correlates with cerebrospinal fluid amine metabolites. Psychiatry Res 1:131–139, 1979

Brown GL, Ebert MH, Goyer PF, et al: Aggression, suicide, and serotonin: relationships to CSF amine metabolites. Am J Psychiatry 139:741–746, 1982

Castellanos FX, Elia J, Kruesi MJP, et al: Cerebrospinal fluid monoamine metabolites in boys with attention deficit hyperactivity disorder. Psychiatry Res 52:305–316, 1994

Christiansen KO: Threshold of tolerance in various population groups illustrated by results from Danish criminological twin study, in Ciba

Foundation Symposium on the Mentally Abnormal Offender. Edited by deReuck AVS, Porter R. London, J&A Churchill, Ltd, 1968, pp 107–116

Christiansen KO: A review of studies of criminality among twins, in Biosocial Basis of Criminal Behavior. Edited by Mednick SA, Christiansen KO. New York, Gardner, 1977, pp 45–80

Cloninger CR, Sigvardsson S, Bohman M, et al: Predisposition to petty criminality in Swedish adoptees, II: crossfostering analysis of gene-environment interaction. Arch Gen Psychiatry 39:1242–1247, 1982

Coccaro EF: Impulsive aggression and central serotonergic system function in humans: an example of a dimensional brain-behavioral relationship. Int Clin Psychopharmacol 7:3–12, 1992

Coccaro EF: Neurotransmitter correlates of impulsive aggression in humans. Ann N Y Acad Sci 794:82–89, 1996

Coccaro EF, Kavoussi RJ: The neuropsychopharmacologic challenge in biological psychiatry. Clin Chemistry 40:319–327, 1994

Coccaro EF, Siever LJ, Klar HM, et al: Serotonergic studies in affective and personality disorder: correlates with suicidal and impulsive aggressive behavior. Arch Gen Psychiatry 46:587–599, 1989

Coccaro EF, Gabriel S, Siever LJ: Buspirone challenge: preliminary evidence for a role for 5-HT-1a receptors in impulsive aggressive behavior in humans. Psychopharmacol Bull 26:393–405, 1990

Coccaro EF, Kavoussi RJ, Hauger RL: Physiologic responses to d-fenfluramine and ipsapirone challenge correlate with indices of aggression in males with personality disorder. Int Clin Psychopharmacol 10:177–180, 1995

Coccaro EF, Kavoussi RJ, Berman ME, et al: Relationship of prolactin response to d-fenfluramine to behavioral and questionnaire assessments of aggression in personality disordered males. Biol Psychiatry 40:157–164, 1996a

Coccaro EF, Kavoussi RJ, Sheline YI, et al: Impulsive aggression in personality disorder: correlates with ^{3}H-paroxetine binding in the platelet. Arch Gen Psychiatry 53:531–536, 1996b

Coccaro EF, Kavoussi RJ, Hauger RL, et al: CSF vasopressin: correlates with indices of aggression and serotonin function in personality disordered subjects. Abstracts of the 35th annual meeting of the American College of Neuropsychopharmacology, p 243, San Juan, Puerto Rico, 1996c

Coccaro EF, Bergeman CS, Kavoussi RJ, et al: Heritability of aggression and irritability: a twin study of the Buss-Durkee aggression scales in adult male subjects. Biol Psychiatry 41:273–284, 1997a

Coccaro EF, Kavoussi RJ, Cooper TB, et al: Central serotonin and aggression: inverse relationship with prolactin response to d-fenfluramine, but not with CSF 5-HIAA concentration in human subjects. Am J Psychiatry 154:1430–1435, 1997b

Coccaro EF, Kavoussi RJ, Sheline YI, et al: Impulsive aggression in personality disorder: correlates with ^{125}I-LSD binding in the platelet. Neuropsychopharmacology 16:211–216, 1997c

Cook EH, Fletcher KE, Wainwright M, et al: Primary structure of the human platelet serotonin 5-HT-2a receptor: identity with frontal cortex serotonin 5-HT-2a receptor. J Neurochemistry 63:465–469, 1994

Crowe RR: Adoption study of antisocial personality disorder. Arch Gen Psychiatry 31:785–791, 1974

Dalgard OS, Kringlen E: A Norwegian twin study of criminality. Br J Criminology 16:213–232, 1976

Delva NJ, Matthews DR, Cowen PJ: Brain serotonin (5-HT) neuroendocrine function in patients taking cholesterol-lowering drugs. Biol Psychiatry 39:100–106, 1996

Delville Y, Mansour KM, Ferris CF: Serotonin blocks vasopressin-facilitated offensice aggression: interactions within the ventrolateral hypothalamus of golden hamsters. Physiol Behav 59:813–816, 1996

Denno DW: Legal implications of genetics and crime research, in Genetics of Criminal and Antisocial Behavior (Ciba Foundation Symposium). Chichester, Wiley, 1996, pp 248–264

Essman WB: Drug effects upon aggressive behavior, in Aggression and Violence: A Psychobiological and Clincial Approach. Edited by Valzelli I, Morgese I. Edizioni Saint Vincent: edizioni Centro Cultrale E congressi Saint Vincent, 1981, pp 150–175

Ferris CF, Delville Y: Vasopressin and serotonin interactions in the control of agonistic behavior. Psychoneuroendocrinology 19:593–601, 1994

Fishbein DH, Lozovsky D, Jaffe JH: Impulsivity, aggression, and neuroendocrine responses to serotonergic stimulation in substance abusers. Biol Psychiatry 25:1049–1066, 1989

Frey T: Electroencephalographic findings in 27 cases with XYY chromosomal pattern and in controls in males with Double Chromosomes. Edited by Forssman H, Wahlstrom J, Wallin L, Akesson HO. Gothenberg, Scandinavian University Books, 1975, pp 55–69

Gardner DL, Lucas PB, Cowdry RW: CSF metabolites in borderline personality disorder compared with normal controls. Biol Psychiatry 28:247–254, 1990

Groesbeck D, D'Asaro B, Nigro C: Polyamine levels in jail inmates. J Orthomol Psychiatry 4:149–152, 1975

Halperin JM, Sharma V, Siever LJ, et al: Serotonergic function in aggressive and nonaggressive boys with attention deficit hyperactivity disorder. Am J Psychiatry 151:243–248, 1994

Halperin JM, Newcorn JH, Schwartz ST, et al: Age-related changes in the association between serotonergic function and aggression in boys with ADHD. Biol Psychiatry 41:682–689, 1997

Hamerton JL: Human population cytogenetics: dilemmas and problems. Am J Hum Genet 28:107–122, 1976

Handelsman L, Holloway K, Kahn RS, et al: Hostility is associated with a low prolactin response to meta-chlorophenylpiperazine in abstinent alcoholics. Alcohol Clin Exp Res 20:824–829, 1996

Higley JD, Mehlman PT, Taub DM, et al: Cerebrospinal fluid monoamine and adrenal correlates of aggression in free-ranging rhesus monkeys. Arch Gen Psychiatry 49:436–441, 1992

Hunter H: XYY males. Br J Psychiatry 131:468–477, 1977

Hutchings B, Mednick SA: Biological and adoptive fathers of male criminal adoptees, in Major Issues in Juvenile Delinquency. Copenhagen, World Health Organization, pp 47–60, 1973

Kaplan JR, Shively CA, Fontenot MB, et al: Demonstration of an association among dietary cholesterol, central serotonergic activity, and social behavior in monkeys. Psychosom Med 56:479–484, 1994

Kruesi MJ, Rapoport JL, Hamberger S, et al: Cerebrospinal fluid metabolites, aggression, and impulsivity in disruptive behavior disorders of children and adolescents. Arch Gen Psychiatry 47:419–462, 1990

Lesch K-P, Wolozin BL, Murphy DL, et al: Primary structure of the human platelet serotonin uptake site: identity with the brain serotonin transporter. J Neurochemistry 60:2319–2322, 1993

Limson R, Goldman D, Roy A, et al: Personality and cerebrospinal fluid monoamine metabolites in alcoholics and controls. Arch Gen Psychiatry 48:437–441, 1991

Linnoila M, Virkkunen M, Scheinin M, et al: Low cerebrospinal fluid 5-hydroxyindolacetic acid concentration differentiates impulsive from nonimpulsive violent behavior. Life Sciences 33:2609–2614, 1983

Linnoila M, DeJong J, Virkkunen M: Family history of alcoholism in violent offenders and alcoholism. Arch Gen Psychiatry 46:613–616, 1989

Lyons MJ: A twin study of self-reported criminal behavior, in Genetics of Criminal and Antisocial Behavior (Ciba Foundation Symposium). Chichester, Wiley, 1995, pp 115–128

Marazziti D, Rotondo A, Presta S, et al: Role of serotonin in human aggressive behavior. Aggressive Behavior 9:347–353, 1993

Mawson AR, Mawson CD: Psychopathy and arousal: a new interpretation of the psychophysiological literature. Biol Psychiatry 12:49–73, 1977

Mehlman PT, Higley JD, Faucher I, et al: Low CSF 5-HIAA concentrations and severe aggression and impaired impulse control in nonhuman primates. Am J Psychiatry 151:1485–1491, 1994

Miles DR, Carey G: Genetic and environmental architecture of human aggression. J Pers Soc Psychol 72:207–217, 1997

Moller SE, Mortensen EL, Breum L, et al: Aggression and personality: association with amino acids and monoamine metabolites. Psychol Med 26:323–331, 1996

Moss HB, Yao JK, Panzak GL: Serotonergic responsivity and behavioral dimensions in antisocial personality disorder with substance abuse. Biol Psychiatry 28:325–338, 1990

Murken JD: The XYY syndrome and Klinefelter's syndrome, in Topics in Human Genetics. Vol 2. Stuttgart, Germany, Georg Thieme, 1973

Nanko S, Saito S, Makino M: X and Y chromatin survey among 1,581 Japanese juvenile delinquents. Japanese J Hum Genet 24:21–25, 1979

Neilson J: Criminality among patients with Klinefelter's syndrome and the XYY syndrome. Br J Psychiatry 117:365–369, 1970

Neilson J, Hendrikson F: Incidence and chromosomal aberrations among males in a Danish youth prison. Acta Psychiatr Scand 48:87–102, 1972

New AS, Trestman RL, Mitroupoulou V, et al: Serotonergic function and self-injurious behavior in personality disorder patients. Psychiatry Res 69:17–26, 1997

New AS, Gelernter J, Yovell Y, et al: Tryptophan hydroxylase genotype is associated with impulsive aggression measures: a preliminary study. Am J Hum Genet (in press)

Nielsen DA, Goldman D, Virkkunen M, et al: Suicidality and 5-hydroxyindoleacetic acid concentration associated with a tryptophan hydroxylase polymorphism. Arch Gen Psychiatry 51:34–38, 1994

Nikkila EA, Taskinen MR: Ethanol-induced alterations of glucose tolerance, postglucose hypoglycemia, and insulin secretion in normal, obese, and diabetic subjects. Diabetes 24:933–943, 1975

Noel B, Benezech M: YY syndrome in French security settings. Clin Genet 12:314, 1977

O'Keane V, Moloney E, O'Neill H, et al: Blunted prolactin responses to d-fenfluramine in sociopathy: evidence for subsensitivity of central serotonergic function. Br J Psychiatry 160:643–646, 1992

O'Keefe SJD, Marks V: Lunchtime gin and tonic a cause of reactive hypoglycemia. Lancet 1:1286–1288, 1977

Pine DS, Coplan JD, Wasserman GA, et al: Neuroendocrine response to d,l-fenfluramine challenge in boys: associations with aggressive behavior and adverse rearing. Arch Gen Psychiatry 54:839–846, 1997

Schiavi RC, Theilgaard A, Owen DR, et al: Sex chromosome anomalies, hormones and aggressivity. Arch Gen Psychiatry 41:93–99, 1984

Sheard M, Marini J, Bridges C, et al: The effect of lithium on impulsive aggressive behavior in man. Am J Psychiatry 133:1409–1413, 1976

Siever L, Trestman RL: The serotonin system and aggressive personality disorder. Int Clin Psychopharmacol 8 (suppl 2):33–39, 1993

Stein DJ, Trestman RL, Mitroupoulou V, et al: Impulsivity and serotonergic function in compulsive personality disorder. J Neuropsychiatry Clin Neurosci 8:393–398, 1996

Stoff DM, Pollock L, Vitiello B, et al: Reduction of ^{3}H-imipramine binding sites on platelets of conduct disordered children. Neuropsychopharmacology 1:55–62, 1987

Stoff DM, Pastiempo AP, Yeung JH, et al: Neuroendocrine responses to
challenge with d,l-fenfluramine and aggression in disruptive behavior disorders of children and adolescents. Psychiatry Res 43:263–276,
1992

Terao T, Yoshimura R, Ohmori O, et al: Effect of serum cholesterol levels
on meta-chlorophenylpiperazine-evoked neuroendocrine responses
in healthy subjects. Biol Psychiatry 41:974–978, 1997

Virkkunen M: Serum cholesterol in antisocial personality. Neuropsychobiology 5:27–30, 1979

Virkkunen M: Reactive hypoglycemic tendency among habitually violent offenders. Neuropsychobiology 8:35–40, 1982

Virkkunen M: Insulin secretion during the glucose tolerance test in antisocial personality. Br J Psychiatry 142:598–604, 1983a

Virkkunen M: Serum cholesterol levels in homicide offenders. Neuropsychobiology 10:65–69, 1983b

Virkkunen M: Reactive hypoglycemic tendency among arsonists. Acta
Psychiatr Scand 69:445–452, 1984

Virkkunen M: Urinary free cortisol secretion in habitually violent offenders. Acta Psychiatr Scand 72:40–44, 1985

Virkkunen M, Huttunen MO: Evidence for abnormal glucose tolerance
test among violent offenders. Neuropsychobiology 8:30–34, 1982

Virkkunen M, Nuutila A, Goodwin FK, et al: Cerebrospinal fluid monoamine metabolite levels in male arsonists. Arch Gen Psychiatry
44:241–247, 1987

Virkkunen M, DeJong J, Bartko J, et al: Relationship of psychobiological
variables to recidivism in violent offenders and impulsive fire setters. Arch Gen Psychiatry 46:600–603, 1989a

Virkkunen M, DeJong J, Bartko J, et al: Psychobiological concomitants
of history of suicide attempts among violent offenders and impulsive fire setters. Arch Gen Psychiatry 46:604–606, 1989b

Virkkunen M, Rawlings R, Tokola R, et al: CSF biochemistries, glucose
metabolism, and diurnal activity rhythms in alcoholic, violent offenders, fire setters, and healthy volunteers. Arch Gen Psychiatry
51:20–27, 1994

Virkkunen M, Eggert, Rawlings R, et al: A prospective follow-up study
of alcoholic violent offenders and fire setters. Arch Gen Psychiatry
53:523–529, 1996

Wetzler S, Kahn RS, Asnis GM, et al: Serotonin receptor sensitivity and
aggression. Psychiatry Res 37:271–279, 1991

Witken HA, Mednick SA, Schulsinger F, et al: Criminality in XYY and XXY men. Science 193:547–555, 1976

Yarura-Tobias JA, Neziroglu FA: Violent behavior, brain dysrhythmia, and glucose dysfunction: a new syndrome. J Orthomol Psychiatry 4:182–188, 1975

Chapter 5

Psychopathology, Crime, and Law

Paul S. Appelbaum, M.D.

As knowledge grows about the roots of human actions, it becomes increasingly possible to identify abnormalities of brain function that appear to underlie some of the more deviant forms of behavior, including violence. Often, these abnormalities are tied to biological causes: genetic influences, psychophysiologic perturbations, neurochemical imbalances, and the like (Mednick et al. 1987). Even when nonbiological causative agents are at work, however, such as poorly titrated environmental stimulation in a child's early development, it is clear that they too are mediated by biological mechanisms; that is the consequence of the brain being an irreducibly biological organ (Searle 1995). The preceding chapters in this book provide ample evidence of the advances being made in determining the relationship of violent criminal behavior to psychopathology and to possibly pathogenic social and biological factors.

My goal in this chapter is not to critique these findings per se—although it is only fair to point out that the search for biological causes of deviant, especially criminal, behavior has had a long and rather unhappy history (Gottfredson and Hirschi 1990). Whether or not the current data ultimately are validated, however, it seems reasonable to assume that at some point we will be able to identify some of the individual-level causes involved in violent criminal behavior, and of necessity they will have biological components. The question of what the implications of such findings may be for the criminal law, now or later,

This work was supported by the Center for Advanced Study in the Behavioral Sciences' Foundations Fund for Research in Psychiatry and NSF Grant #SBR-9022192.

is therefore inescapable. I focus in this chapter particularly on the law of criminal responsibility, which is usually subsumed in the popular mind under the rubric of the "insanity defense," but I also address some considerations of correctional practice.

How might data on the psychopathological roots of at least some criminal behavior affect the law? One response might be for the law to shift its approach to determining the culpability of persons who commit criminal acts. Our legal tradition has long made exceptions to the general rules of the criminal law, allowing certain mentally ill persons who commit crimes to avoid punishment. Such persons are denoted "legally insane" and are not held responsible for their acts. Instead of putting them in prisons, we put them in hospitals; rather than punishing them, we treat them; instead of holding them until their sentences expire, we allow them to return to the community as soon as their disorder is under sufficient control that they are no longer likely to be dangerous.

Perhaps, it might be argued, this will become the societal response to criminal activity in general, or at least to the actions of those subgroups of criminals (e.g., recidivistic criminal offenders [Raine 1993], or those with low CNS serotonin levels [Virkkunen et al. 1994]) whose behavior appears to be symptomatic of their psychopathology. They will be exculpated from responsibility for their acts—since their disordered brains played a causal role—and confined only so long as they require secure treatment.

A second possibility is somewhat less radical but would require an equally profound attitudinal change in the criminal justice system. Since we do not now have effective treatments for most criminals (i.e., interventions that will substantially reduce the rate of offending in the future), we might at the least reorient the punitive aspects of our reaction to them. Adrian Raine exemplifies this approach in his recent book:

> Perhaps, at the least, such individuals should not be punished as harshly as they currently are. One scenario would be to place offenders deemed to be disordered into institutions that are fully secure . . . but which allow as much freedom as possible given the

constraints of keeping such offenders away from society, at the same time minimizing all punitive aspects of the regime . . . such an environment would attempt to cultivate new treatment programs based on experimental research into treatment interventions. . . . (1993, p. 308)

I am somewhat skeptical, however, that either of these events will come to pass. I do not believe that—even with more substantial data than we have today—the law will soon evidence a willingness to exculpate repeated offenders whose behavior appears "symptomatic" of an underlying disorder of the brain, or that it will countenance a radical transformation of the correctional system toward a focus on therapy rather than punishment. Moreover, I am inclined to believe that the law would be correct in taking these positions. To explain why, we must explore the law's traditional approach to mental disorder and crime.

diffe over time

Legal Views of Mental Disorder and Crime

A brief survey of how the law has dealt with the relationship between crime and mental disorder leads us back to antiquity, when the moral intuition first appeared that a person's mental state might preclude punishment for a crime. Aristotle argued in his *Nichomachean Ethics* that confusion over the reality of a situation—perhaps a person's delusional belief that he or she was being harmed by another—might provide a moral excuse for persons who acted unlawfully in response to those beliefs (Aristotle 1962). Aristotle's contentions, however, had little impact on his Greek contemporaries, who punished perpetrators irrespective of their underlying motives or beliefs—a form of strict liability for criminal acts. Roman law, in contrast, seems to have inclined toward leniency regarding those who acted under the influence of madness—albeit less on the basis of concerns about moral blameworthiness than on the grounds that such unfortunates had already been punished by fate, and it was not for man to add to their afflictions (Walker 1985).

Aristotle's conception of the moral significance of one's motivation, though ignored in most criminal law systems of antiquity and the Middle Ages, was embraced by the Church in its canon law. Kept alive in this way, Aristotelian concepts of culpability entered the Anglo-American legal tradition through the writings of the thirteenth-century jurist Bracton, who asserted that a culpable mental state (or *mens rea*) was a necessary component of criminal culpability. "A crime is not committed," he wrote, "unless the will to harm be present" (Bracton 1968). This formulation, in theory, excluded from moral and legal guilt all persons who caused harm unintentionally, including those who may have intended to commit certain acts but did not understand their wrongfulness. Although initially a finding that the defendant had committed a criminal act but lacked *mens rea* was considered a conviction—with avoidance of punishment dependent on a pardon from the Crown—by the beginning of the sixteenth-century juries had acquired the power to acquit such defendants outright (Walker 1968).

Tests of Criminal Responsibility

The subsequent four centuries in England and America alike have been marked by a search for precisely the right formulation to characterize those persons who should not be held responsible for their acts. These have evolved along a spectrum of rigor. Early formulations such as the "wild beast test" (the defendant did "not know what he was doing, no more than an infant, than a brute or wild beast" [*Rex v. Arnold* 1723]) required total behavioral dyscontrol and utter detachment from reality—often referred to as "furious," "frenzied," or "raving" madness. Not many defendants would be expected to meet this standard, and the historical evidence suggests that it was abandoned in practice well before the start of the nineteenth century, to which its demise is usually dated (Walker 1968). It is echoed today in those American states (Idaho, Montana, and Utah) that have abolished a special defense of insanity, exculpating only those defendants

who demonstrate that they lack *mens rea* in the classical sense—
that is, they truly were unaware of the nature of their acts.

In the seventeenth and eighteenth centuries, a new test gained
ascendance; it required the defendant to prove that he or she
lacked the ability to distinguish between good and evil. This
approach was epitomized by the *McNaughtan* standard, formally
adopted in England in 1843: A defendant could be exculpated if
"at the time of the committing of the act, the party accused was
laboring under such a defect of reason, from disease of the mind,
as not to know the nature and quality of the act he was doing;
or, if he did know it, that he did not know he was doing what
was wrong" (Moran 1981). *McNaughtan* remains the law in England to this day, and it was rapidly adopted by many jurisdictions in the United States. It epitomizes Bracton's dictum that the
"will to harm"—that is, a knowledge that one is doing something wrong—is an absolute prerequisite to criminal culpability.

In nineteenth-century America, another test gained in popularity, often added to the *McNaughtan* standard: the "irresistible
impulse" test. It dealt with persons who may have known that
they were committing a wrongful act but felt powerless to stop
themselves from doing so (Goldstein 1967). The idea of irresistible impulses fits well with contemporary notions of "moral insanity," a corruption of the moral senses, arguably akin to what
today would be considered an antisocial personality. Persons
with affective disorders, more so than those with disorders on
the schizophrenic spectrum, are at least in principle more likely
to benefit from the irresistible impulse standard.

Innovations in the twentieth century have been modest. The
McNaughtan "right from wrong" test has been combined in a
modified form with the irresistible impulse test in the widely
adopted American Law Institute (ALI) formulation. Until recently, this was the dominant test of legal insanity in the United
States:

A person is not responsible for criminal conduct if at the time of
such conduct as a result of mental disease or defect he lacks substantial capacity to appreciate the criminality [wrongfulness] of
his conduct or to conform his conduct to the requirements of the
law. (American Law Institute 1955)

More recently there has been a trend to discard the irresistible impulse portion of the ALI standard, in the belief that it provides too much leeway for defendants to avoid punishment (Appelbaum 1994). A brief experiment also occurred in the District of Columbia with a standard first proposed in nineteenth-century New Hampshire, which exculpated defendants if they merely showed that their criminal behavior was the product of their mental illness, regardless of their cognitive knowledge of wrongfulness or their volitional controls (*Durham v. U.S.* 1954). This approach was abandoned after a few years, in large part because of its indeterminacy (*U.S. v. Brawner* 1972), but we shall return to consider the lesson taught by this episode momentarily.

Implications of the Legal Formulations of Nonculpability

What do all of these approaches have in common? Each standard has been used by the law to reflect a moral consensus that some people are so disordered that they should not be held responsible for their behavior. The issue, then, is moral, not scientific or medical, or even narrowly legal. The standards focus on a small group of people—in most cases people who were psychotic at the time of their crimes—the exceptions to the general rule that people will be punished for their criminal acts. Recent data indicate that the insanity plea is considered seriously in under 1% of felony cases, and that it is successful in no more than one-fourth of the cases in which it is used (Steadman et al. 1993). The history of the insanity defense has shown us that when any standard threatens to be applied so broadly as to include more than a minuscule percentage of the most severely affected offenders, that standard is rejected in favor of a more restrictive rule. This is what happened with the "product of mental illness" test in the District of Columbia, and in the reforms following John F. Hinckley, Jr.'s, successful use of the insanity defense after his attempt on President Reagan's life (Steadman et al. 1993).

Moreover, the application of the insanity defense is highly dependent on the degree of moral outrage the defendant's crime evokes in the general population (Finkel 1996). This has been the case for as long as we have records of insanity defense trials (Walker 1968). Even extremely psychotic defendants will be convicted for their actions if their behavior is sufficiently heinous. Both "Son of Sam," whose dog allegedly told him to commit the murders he perpetrated on a lovers' lane in Queens, New York, and, more recently, Jeffrey Dahmer, who ate his victims after he killed them, were found guilty despite behavior that bespoke severe mental disorder. The same is true for John Salvi, who killed two people in attacks on Boston area abortion clinics and committed suicide after his conviction. When this rule is violated, as it was in John F. Hinckley, Jr.'s, acquittal, the greatest pressure arises for abolition of the insanity defense.

When the time has come for the law to formulate its standards for judging criminal responsibility, lack of blameworthiness has most often been associated with an inability to recognize the wrongfulness of one's acts. The underlying rationale, in oversimplified form, appears to be that persons who cannot distinguish between right and wrong are in no position to make meaningful choices regarding their behavior, and therefore it would be unfair to punish them for the consequences of their actions (Bonnie 1983). Less commonly, exculpation has been extended to those persons who may have known their acts were wrong but lacked sufficient behavioral controls to stop themselves from performing those acts. This category of impaired offender is a controversial one, in part because we know so little about matters of will. At what point, for example, do we say that a person has no longer chosen to act the way he or she did, but instead has been compelled by some inner force (American Psychiatric Association 1982)? This debate will be familiar to everyone who has followed the literature on alcoholism (Fingarette 1988), and the argument can be extended to other forms of addiction or compulsive behavior.

Finally, although it is not apparent from this brief review of the insanity defense, it is important to recognize that for much of its modern history, a verdict of not guilty by reason of insanity resulted in a Pyrrhic victory for the defendant. Since the turn of the nineteenth century, defendants who ostensibly have been ex-culpated for their criminal actions have been subject afterward to indefinite confinement in psychiatric facilities (Moran 1985). That confinement was often lifelong. When legal developments resulted in more frequent release of insanity acquittees in the last several decades, we again saw pressure to tighten the standards for acquittal, or to abolish the defense (LaFond and Durham 1992). More creatively, several states now extend supervision of insanity acquittees in the community, endowing oversight boards with the power to reconfine acquittees at the first sign of noncompliance with treatment conditions or an increased risk of recurrent criminal behavior (Bloom and Williams 1994; Mc-Greevy et al. 1991; Scott et al. 1990; Spodak et al. 1984; Wieder-anders 1992). Exculpation is a moral judgment, but its practical consequences have not been great. The average insanity acquit-tee serves as long or longer in confinement than a defendant who is convicted of the same charges (Steadman 1985).

The Law's Response to the Psychopathologizing of Crime

With this background, we can now consider how the law is likely to respond to claims that many forms of criminal behavior, es-pecially violent and recidivistic behavior, are, in reality, forms of psychopathology, based in dysfunction of the brain. The intrinsic rationale for the insanity defense, as I have noted, has been the unfairness of punishing people who cannot make meaningful choices about their behavior—usually because they have a sub-stantial absence of the ability to recognize the wrongfulness of their acts. Even taking as proven the assertions that many of-fenders, especially serious recidivists, suffer from a variety of neurobiological deficits, there is as yet no evidence to suggest that these deficits substantially impair the ability to recognize that criminal actions are generally considered to be wrong.

Psychopaths, criminals who commit repetitive violent offenses, firesetters, recidivistic sex offenders—the leading categories of offenders for whom purported biological dysfunctions have been identified (Raine 1993; Virkkunen et al. 1989; Wright et al. 1990)—all generally are aware that their acts are viewed as wrongful. As a simple test, few offenders falling into these categories fail to flee the scene of the crime (as do some psychotic offenders [Martell and Dietz 1992]), and most take other measures to avoid detection. Indeed, even proponents of differential treatment for such offenders have not maintained that they do not understand that their actions are subject to punishment. This group, therefore, falls outside the scope of the usual justification for exculpation. Regardless of the abnormalities identified in the functioning of their brains, pointing to the psychopathological roots of their behavior is unlikely, from this perspective, to alter how the courts view their actions.

Of course, it could be argued that the second prong of the modern insanity defense—the irresistible impulse test—is actually more relevant to this group. Rather than failing to understand that their actions are wrong, this argument goes, impaired offenders are simply unable to control their criminal behavior. If, indeed, one of the effects of reduced serotonin levels is to increase impulsivity, and many criminal offenders have low central serotonin (Virkkunen et al. 1994); if psychopathy involves, in part, a reduced ability to delay gratification, and many offenders are psychopaths (Guze 1976); if frontal lobe dysfunction has a negative effect on judgment (Damasio 1994) and stimulates aggression (Grafman et al. 1996), and many offenders show signs of damage to their frontal lobes (Elliott 1992); then the actions of these offenders may derive from impaired volitional controls on behavior. Should the law not recognize this problem?

The irresistible impulse test, it will be recalled, was one of the last standards introduced for legal insanity, and when public dissatisfaction with the insanity defense has been manifest, it has been the first element to be sacrificed (Steadman et al. 1993). Volitional control is so difficult to measure, particularly retrospectively, and the concept itself is so imprecise, that the law has always felt, at a minimum, a good deal of ambivalence about utilizing the irresistible impulse standard. So grounding the argument here puts it on the weakest possible foundation, from a legal perspective.

When the irresistible impulse standard has been employed, however, it has generally required profound deficits in the ability to control one's actions. The most liberal version of the test has been whether a defendant lacks *substantial* capacity to conform his or her behavior to the requirements of the law. In practice, the "policeman at the elbow" test is often the touchstone at trial: Would the defendant have committed the act in question if a policeman had been at his or her elbow? If so, the impulse was truly irresistible; if not, the defendant was capable of at least some degree of control, should have exercised it here, and deserves to be convicted. Even if the degree of impulsivity manifest by repetitive offenders, firesetters, and other classes of offenders is substantial, it is unlikely that many—if any—of them would meet a test of this degree of rigor. Thus, the law is not likely to alter its treatment of them from this perspective either.

Yet a third point might be argued, as Adrian Raine does in his recent book (1993). Because of the concatenation of events beyond their control, many of the serious recidivists with whom he is concerned, Raine maintains, even if they do not meet the classical tests for legal insanity, cannot be said to be exercising a substantial degree of free will when they commit their criminal acts. Prenatal injuries, maternal deprivation, poor nutrition, physical and sexual abuse, head injury, educational failure and the like all made these people what they are today. They had no control over these influences; their free will, if not absent, is at least impaired; "the implication is that criminal offenders should not be punished as severely as they are currently for their actions" (Raine 1993, p. 312).

The problem with this argument, of course, is that the same thing could be said about any of us. We are all the result of a complex set of interactions between environmental and biological factors. All of us do what we do, in large part, because of those influences. Thus, when any of us break the law—as we all do at some time or another—it is because of who we are and who we have been, from prenatal environment, through childhood, to the present. What criminal could not claim that his or her actions were not substantially the product of free will (Morris 1982)? So defined, the concept of free will is all but meaningless. It is precisely once the historical, biological, and environmental variables are factored in that free will, such as it is, becomes operative. Criminal punishment is not inconsistent with the recognition of the many factors that influence behavior. But the law assumes that a person will exercise control of his or her behavior despite the variables—ranging from deprivation to temptation to intoxication—that might incline that person to violate the law. Arguments to the contrary are not likely to be persuasive in a court of justice.

My argument to this point, of course, has suggested that the law as it currently stands is unlikely to be interpreted as applicable to nonpsychotic offenders whose behavior appears to have roots in subtle dysfunction of the brain. But perhaps the law will expand its exculpatory reach as new data become available and force the reconceptualization of criminal behavior. There are sound reasons of policy as to why this is unlikely to occur, reasons that have accounted in large measure for the current shape of the criminal law.

As I noted earlier, the insanity defense and other exculpatory or mitigating strategies have been crafted to apply to only a small percentage of defendants—they are the exceptions that prove the rule that persons will be punished if they commit criminal acts. Expanding the scope of these legal rules has, at a certain point, always led to a backlash in which the previous concessions have been retracted. One need only recall in this regard the furor following the successful "Twinkie defense" of Dan White, the murderer of Mayor Moscone and Supervisor Harvey Milk in San Francisco. The finding that White's actions occurred during a state of diminished capacity (which reduced the degree of criminal culpability, but did not eliminate it entirely, as does the insanity defense), led to a repudiation of the doctrine of diminished capacity in California, the state in which it had found its most fertile soil (Slovenko 1995).

The suggestion that we might excuse the behavior of recidivist criminals, sex offenders, firesetters, and other offenders because their brains may function differently from most of the population would extend the scope of such doctrines well beyond where they have ever reached before. Rather than punishing most criminal acts, we would end up excusing them or mitigating their sanctions. One of the cornerstones of the criminal law is the notion that the prospect of punishment will deter criminal behavior. No nation has ever chosen to undertake a rigorous test of this principle by abolishing its criminal laws. But that might nearly be the effect of imputing exculpatory impact to dysfunctions that affect a large proportion of those who commit criminal acts. This is not to suggest that defense attorneys will not try to use new information about the biological influences on behavior to win exculpation or mitigation for their clients; undoubtedly they will (Morse 1996). But there are good reasons why the insanity defense and related standards have been kept quite narrow. The likely effect of opening the floodgates of exculpatory defenses makes the wisdom of that course evident.

There is a particular irony in the identification of those offenders for whom, by virtue of biological abnormalities of the brain, exculpation is urged: psychopaths, violent recidivists, arsonists, sex offenders. The first two groups commit the majority of serious offenses (Guze 1976; Weiner 1989), and the last two are probably the most feared. Even defendants who might objectively be said to qualify for the insanity defense almost never receive it when their actions pass a certain threshold of public fear or revulsion (Stone 1985). The criminals we are talking about here are those most likely to arouse those emotions in the public at large. This is precisely the group that the public—not without justification—believes deserves the longest sentences and the harshest punishment, from both a retributive and deterrence perspective. It is difficult to conceive of a circumstance in which that perception would be altered.

Finally, in terms of legal response to the latest research findings, if such offenders will not be exculpated, perhaps they could be treated. What about the more modest goal of turning prisons into places of research and therapy rather than of punishment? Although it sounds pleasingly humanitarian, I suggest that the criminal justice and correctional systems will be appropriately wary of this change in emphasis. American psychiatry went through a period of optimism about its abilities to understand and treat criminal behaviors from the 1930s to the early 1950s (Menninger 1966). The result was a variety of treatment programs in prisons and other facilities for repetitive offenders, sex offenders, and others (Group for the Advancement of Psychiatry 1977). Sentencing practices were even altered to allow some of these persons to be held indefinitely until "cure" was attained (Dix 1983; Lindman and McIntyre 1961).

The mental health professions have never been able to document their ability to "treat" criminal behavior, if by treatment we mean to reduce the incidence of recurrence. In part, this has been due to the minimal funding and other support provided to treatment programs, in part to the primitive state of research methods for establishing such conclusions. When studies have been done with selected populations (e.g., sex offenders), however, the results have not been encouraging (Sturgeon and Taylor 1980). As a corollary, mental health professionals have also been unable to determine when prisoners are no longer likely to be dangerous (whether because of their treatment or in spite of it) and are therefore ready to be released (Monahan 1981). These failures have left in their substantial wake an understandable reluctance on the part of criminal justice and correctional officials to put much stock in treatment-oriented approaches. Psychiatrists and other mental health professionals will have to demonstrate convincingly their ability to alter criminal behavior, in those few places where access to correctional populations exists, before the doors of the prisons swing open to new treatment programs. The data needed to support such efforts simply do not exist.

Conclusion

This analysis should not be taken as reflecting a lack of appreciation for the advances that are being made in understanding the correlates of violent criminal behavior, such as are demonstrated in the preceding chapters. If effective prevention and treatment of the predisposition to crime are ever to be possible, it will be due in part to such work. The most potent agent of change in legal approaches to crime is likely to result from the ability of the mental health professions to treat criminal behavior effectively. Biologically oriented investigations should be encouraged, if only for the hope they hold out that this may some day be possible. But I am skeptical, given the current state of knowledge, that biological research into the roots of criminal behavior has anything meaningful to say to the law at present, and I doubt that it will influence the law in the foreseeable future.

References

American Law Institute: Model Penal Code, Sec. 4.01 (1955)

American Psychiatric Association: Statement on the Insanity Defense. Washington, DC, American Psychiatric Association, December 1982

Appelbaum PS: Almost a Revolution: Mental Health Law and the Limits of Change. New York, Oxford University Press, 1994

Aristotle: Nichomachean Ethics, Book Four. Indianapolis, IN, Bobbs-Merrill, 1962

Bloom JD, Williams MH: Management and Treatment of Insanity Acquittees: A Model for the 1990s. Washington, DC, American Psychiatric Press, 1994

Bonnie R: The moral basis of the insanity defense. American Bar Association Journal 69:194–197, 1983

Bracton H: Of the laws and customs of England, cited in Walker N: Crime and Insanity in England, Vol 1: Historical Perspective. Edinburgh, Scotland, Edinburgh University Press, 1968

Damasio AR: Descartes' Error: Emotion, Reason and the Human Brain. New York, Avon Books, 1994

Dix GE: Special dispositional alternatives for abnormal offenders: developments in the law, in Mentally Disordered Offenders: Perspectives From Law and Social Science. Edited by Monahan J, Steadman HJ. New York, Plenum, 1983, pp 133–190

Durham v U.S., 214 F.2d 862 (D.C.Cir. 1954)

Elliott FA: Violence: the neurologic contribution—an overview. Arch Neurol 49:595–603, 1992

Fingarette H: Heavy Drinking: The Myth of Alcoholism as a Disease. Berkeley, CA, University of California Press, 1988

Finkel N: Commonsense Justice. Cambridge, MA, Harvard University Press, 1996

Goldstein AS: The Insanity Defense. New Haven, CT, Yale University Press, 1967

Gottfredson MR, Hirschi T: A General Theory of Crime. Stanford, CA, Stanford University Press, 1990

Grafman J, Schwab K, Warden D, et al: Frontal lobe injuries, violence, and aggression: a report of the Vietnam Head Injury Study. Neurology 46:1231–1238, 1996

Group for the Advancement of Psychiatry: Psychiatry and Sex Psychopath Legislation: The 30s to the 80s. New York, GAP, 1977

Guze SB: Criminality and Psychiatric Disorders. New York, Oxford University Press, 1976

LaFond J, Durham M: Back to the Asylum. New York, Oxford University Press, 1992

Lindman FT, McIntyre DM: The Mentally Disabled and the Law. Chicago, IL, University of Chicago Press, 1961

Martell DA, Dietz PE: Mentally disordered offenders who push or attempt to push victims onto subway tracks in New York City. Arch Gen Psychiatry 49:472–475, 1992

McGreevy MA, Steadman HJ, Dvoskin JA, Dollard N: New York State's system of managing insanity acquittees in the community. Hosp Community Psychiatry 42:512–517, 1991

Mednick SA, Moffitt TE, Stack SA (eds): The Causes of Crime: New Biological Approaches. Cambridge, UK, Cambridge University Press, 1987

Menninger K: The Crime of Punishment. New York, Viking, 1966

Monahan J: The Clinical Prediction of Violent Behavior. Rockville, MD, NIMH, 1981

Moran R: Knowing Right from Wrong: The Insanity Defense of Daniel McNaughtan. New York, Free Press, 1981

Moran R: The modern foundations for the insanity defense: the cases of James Hadfield (1800) and Daniel McNaughtan (1843), in The Insanity Defense. Edited by Moran R. Ann Am Acad Political Soc Sci 477:31–42, 1985

Morris N: Madness and the Criminal Law. Chicago, IL, University of Chicago Press, 1982

Morse SJ: Brain and blame. Georgetown Law Journal 84:527–549, 1996

Raine A: The Psychopathology of Crime. San Diego, CA, Academic Press, 1993

Rex v Arnold, 16 How.St.Tr. 684 (1723)

Scott DC, Zonana HV, Geta MA: Monitoring insanity acquittees: Connecticut's PSRB. Hosp Community Psychiatry 41:980–984, 1990

Searle JR: The Rediscovery of the Mind. Cambridge, MA, MIT Press, 1995

Slovenko R: Psychiatry and Criminal Culpability. New York, Wiley, 1995

Spodak MK, Silver SB, Wright CU: Criminality of discharged insanity acquittees: fifteen-year experience in Maryland reviewed. Bull Am Acad Psychiatry Law 12:373–382, 1984

Steadman HJ: Empirical research on the insanity defense, in The Insanity Defense. Edited by Moran R. Ann Am Acad Political Soc Sci 477:58–71, 1985

Steadman HJ, McGreevy MA, Morrissey JP, et al: Before and After Hinckley: Evaluating Insanity Defense Reform. New York, Guilford, 1993

Stone AA: Law, Psychiatry, and Morality. Washington, DC, American Psychiatric Press, 1985

Sturgeon V, Taylor J: Report of a five-year follow-up study of mentally disordered sex offenders released from Atascadero State Hospital in 1973. Criminal Justice Journal 4:31–64, 1980

U.S. v Brawner, 471 F.2d 969 (D.C.Cir. 1972)

Virkkunen M, DeJong J, Bartko J, et al: Relationship of psychobiological variables to recidivism in violent offenders and impulsive firesetters. Arch Gen Psychiatry 46:600–603, 1989

Virkkunen M, Rawlings R, Tokola R, et al: CSF biochemistries, glucose metabolism, and diurnal activity rhythms in alcoholic, violent offenders, fire setters, and healthy volunteers. Arch Gen Psychiatry 51:20–27, 1994

Walker N: Crime and Insanity in England, Vol 1: Historical Perspective. Edinburgh, Scotland, Edinburgh University Press, 1968

Walker N: The insanity defense before 1800, in The Insanity Defense. Edited by Moran R. Ann Am Acad Political Soc Sci 477:25–30, 1985

Wiederanders MR: Recidivism of disordered offenders who were conditionally vs. unconditionally released. Behav Sci Law 10:141–148, 1992

Weiner NA: Violent criminal careers and "violent career criminals," in Violent Crime, Violent Criminals. Edited by Weiner NA, Wolfgang ME. Newbury Park, CA, Sage Publications, 1989

Wright P, Nobrega J, Langevin R, et al: Brain density and symmetry in pedophilic and sexually aggressive offenders. Ann Sex Res 3:319–328, 1990

Afterword

Andrew E. Skodol, M.D.

In his 1993 book entitled *The Psychopathology of Crime: Criminal Behavior as a Clinical Disorder,* Adrian Raine (1993) argues that individuals who commit repeated criminal acts suffer from psychopathology, whether or not they exhibit the signs and symptoms of clinical disorders currently classified in official nosologies. In other words, Raine contends that criminality meets currently accepted *general* criteria for the concept of psychopathology and, thus, is by definition a mental disorder. He argues that criminality and psychopathology are both abnormal in that they 1) represent deviations from statistical norms (i.e., are relatively infrequent), from ideals of mental health, and from social norms; 2) cause distress or suffering to self or others; 3) lead to impairment in functioning; 4) overlap with behaviors that are indicators of mental disorders already in official classifications; 5) are associated with biological dysfunctions; and 6) meet DSM-III-R (and DSM-IV) general definitions of mental disorder. Whether or not one is persuaded by the voluminous data Raine brings to bear on the equivalence of criminality and psychopathology, the chapters in this book clearly indicate strong links.

Narrow definitions of mental disorder (e.g., schizophrenia and major mood disorders) appear to be associated with an up to fivefold increase in the prevalence of violent behavior in affected persons over persons without mental disorders in the general population. If the definition of mental disorder is appropriately expanded to include alcohol use disorders and other substance use disorders, the prevalence of violent behavior among affected persons increases to between 12 and 16 times that among the unaffected. Including Axis II personality disorders, as yet not well studied, with the exception of antisocial personality disorder (ASPD), should eventually be shown to further increase the risk of violence in community populations. As Widiger and Trull (1994) point out, aggression or violence is a defining feature of antisocial and borderline personality disorders (BPD), and hostile, antagonistic traits are exhibited by persons with 7 of the 10 DSM-IV Axis II disorders, including paranoid, schizotypal, antisocial, borderline, histrionic, narcissistic, and obsessive-compulsive personality disorders. Antisocial personality disorder is overrepresented in studies of mental disorders in prisoners (as reviewed by Beck and Wencel), and ASPD or psychopathy has been found to be present among hospitalized schizophrenic patients who commit violent offenses. In the study reported in this book by Coid, it is readily apparent that if other personality disorders are sought in criminal populations, substantial rates will be found. Axis II disorders, especially ASPD and BPD, would also likely contribute to the genesis of violent behavior, due to the increased risk of developing substance use disorders to people with these two personality disorders.

How dangerous are people with mental disorders? Again, starting with the narrowest definition of disorder, the vast majority (90%) of persons with schizophrenia or major mood disorder do not commit violence. Furthermore, there seems to be little support for the popular misconception that individuals with major mental disorders strike at random. Rather, their violent acts appear to be directed at close family members and significant others. A larger proportion of persons with alcohol (25%) or other substance use disorders (35%) commit violent acts, but they are still a minority. In the case of persons with ASPD, however, given that aggressiveness is a core feature, a majority of affected persons would be expected to have a history of violent behavior. Increasing attention is being paid to the aggressive potential of patients with BPD; preliminary indications are that 40%–50% of patients seen *outside* of a forensic setting will report assaultive and other aggressive acts (Skodol et al. 1996).

What proportion of violence in society can be attributed to mental disorder? Major mental disorders have a relatively low prevalence in the population. The Epidemiologic Catchment Area (ECA) Study (Robins and Regier 1991) and the National

Comorbidity Survey (NCS) (Kessler et al. 1994) estimate lifetime prevalences of schizophrenia and other nonaffective psychotic disorders at 0.7%–1.5%, bipolar disorder at 0.8%–1.6%, and major depression at 4.9%–17.1%. Thus, restricting the proportion of U.S. crime to approximately 10% of a population of at most 20% (and possibly less than 7%) yields low estimates of the contribution of mental disorder to violence in America. Lifetime substance use disorders (including alcoholism) have been estimated to be present in 20%–35.4% of the population, based on these two epidemiologic surveys, and ASPD at 2.6%–3.5%. No other personality disorders were formally assessed in either the ECA or the NCS studies, but other nonpatient samples have indicated that 10%–18% of the population suffers from some type of Axis II disorder (Skodol 1997). Since larger proportions of patients with substance use disorders or personality disorders commit acts of violence, these figures suggest that the contribution of mental illness, more broadly defined, to the problem of violent crime is not as trivial as it would seem at first glance.

In addition, the boundaries of categorical diagnoses of mental disorders are somewhat arbitrary. DSM-IV has a relatively limited set of formal diagnoses for disorders characterized by violent behavior—antisocial personality disorder, intermittent explosive disorder, conduct disorder in children and adolescents, and several of the paraphilias. Aggressiveness, however, is a universal personality trait on which all humans vary. Thus, the studies conducted and reported by Coccaro and associates of the heritability of aggression and of the neurotransmitter, metabolic, and hormonal mediators of aggression are applicable across the range of distribution of the trait of aggression, and not simply to the pathological groups studied initially. In that there is evidence of a continuous distribution of biological abnormalities across a spectrum of aggressive behaviors and similarities in findings between traditionally "disordered" groups and "nondisordered" aggressive groups, the clear-cut distinction between disorder and no disorder becomes blurred. Therefore, according to a dimensional definition of "disordered aggression," the role of "disorder" in the genesis of violent crime might actually become quite large.

How should the judicial and penal systems respond to the findings that link violent crime and mental disorder or that document an underlying biological dysfunction? Appelbaum clearly presents the reality that the courts serve the public welfare and that the more the public is faced with the gruesome acts one human being can perpetrate against another, the less they want to be confronted with these possibilities. Thus, media's playing up to violent crime ("if it bleeds, it leads") helps to fuel public fear and revulsion, leading to stiffer sentences for criminals, growing jail populations, expanding budgets for prisons, and so forth. But public reaction aside, current legal definitions of criminal responsibility as embodied by the American Law Institute formulation, that is, "lacking substantial capacity to appreciate the wrongfulness of his conduct," would not apply to the vast majority of violent criminals with mental disorders. Therefore, more generously determined exculpation from responsibility for crimes because of their link to mental disorder seems unlikely to result from these new findings for several reasons. And without better data indicating the efficacy of treatments for mental disorders, especially substance use disorders and personality disorders, that curtail associated criminal behavior, it seems unlikely that prisons in this country will be converted to hospitals.

What then is the role of the psychiatrist in helping society cope with violence, if violence is found increasingly on phenomenological or biological grounds to indicate emotional disturbance? The answer would seem to be predicated on the causes of violence in the mentally ill.

The studies on the crucial role of threatening delusions in the genesis of violent behavior in psychotic persons point to the role of antipsychotic medications in controlling delusional thinking, and consequently reducing violence, in the small segment of the criminally violent population suffering from psychotic disorders. If it is true, as Beck and McNamee report, that a well-maintained medication regimen renders a violent psychotic person no more dangerous than an ordinary person, then strategies for getting more patients into treatment and ensuring their continuing compliance with treatment need to be further developed. Better-tolerated antipsychotic drugs should be developed, more open access to treatment ensured, better monitoring of patients implemented, and more supportive and stable living situations (i.e., not the street) provided.

For alcohol and other drug-abusing and dependent persons, effective treatments are being sought. Their impact on reducing violence associated with substance use remains to be seen. Treatment compliance is an issue. But contextual and other social factors are also relevant. Personality traits and other psychosocial risk factors for substance abuse and antisociality have much in common. Both share personality traits of impulsivity/disinhibition (Sher and Trull 1994). Families are broken, abusive, or neglectful. Ineffective parental supervision and control reinforce childhood conduct problems, which in turn increase the likelihood of academic failure and association with deviant peer groups and subsequent substance abuse and antisocial behavior (Loeber 1990). Opportunities for scholastic and occupational success and improvement in the conditions of living in adult life often become limited. Without renewal and stabilization of the family, schools, and other institutions in the community, the outlook is bleak. Psychiatrists should come to grips with the need to work as much on prevention of violence as on the development and administration of efficacious treatment for it.

Helping parents deal with the economic stresses and social demands of family life will reduce their potential for abusive or neglectful treatment of their children. Teaching them how to provide for the emotional and educational needs of their children can prepare children to succeed in school and avoid delinquency. Teaching children nonaggressive approaches to conflict resolution at an early age provides them with skills to avert the need for violent behavior. Although preventative efforts cost money, they can be shown to save much more, in terms of the costs of the criminal justice system and the costs to victims of violent behavior (Gibson 1995).

In the realm of the personality disorders, proven treatments may be even harder to find. Some new psychotherapeutic and pharmacologic approaches to the impulsivity of borderline patients have been developed and show promise, but the enthusiasm generated by still relatively sparse data supporting their effectiveness attests to both the great need for better treatment strategies and the relative neglect of this area of psychopathology. When it comes to reducing violent crime in society or preventing it, personality disorders would seem to be prime targets for intervention. For now, detection of personality pathology in violent criminals, delineation of motives, and prognostication based on what is known about the potential for recidivism and the negative prognostic factors in the therapy of severe personality disorders (e.g., maliciousness, contemptuousness, vengefulness, mendacity) (Stone 1992) may be all that psychiatrists can contribute clinically.

Models of violent behavior almost invariably depict a disturbance in the balance between impulse and control (Skodol 1984). Brain damage, psychosis, high aggressivity, sensation seeking, provocation, desperation—all may lead to increased impulsivity. Low IQ, substance intoxication, defective conscience, disintegration of family structure, school failure, delinquent peers, and dissolution of cultural institutions all may contribute to reduced behavioral control. In the recently published initial report from the National Longitudinal Study on Adolescent Health, Resnick et al. (1997) found that parent-family connectedness and school connectedness helped to mitigate against risk factors (including history of victimization and antisocial behavior) for violent behavior among junior high school and high school students. Psychiatrists need to assume responsibility to society as teachers and leaders to help to rectify current trends toward disorganization and instability in social customs and institutions (Millon 1992) in an effort to avoid significant increases in criminal behavior in the future.

References

Gibson CM: A strong community is a safe one. Yale Medicine 30:6–7, 1995

Kessler RC, McGonagle KA, Zhao S, et al: Lifetime and 12-month prevalence of DSM-III-R psychiatric disorders in the United States: results from the National Comorbidity Survey. Arch Gen Psychiatry 51:8–19, 1994

Loeber R: Development and risk factors of juvenile antisocial behavior and delinquency. Clin Psychol Rev 10:1–41, 1990

Millon T: The borderline construct: introductory notes on its history, theory, and empirical grounding, in Borderline Personality Disorder: Clinical and Empirical Perspectives. Edited by Clarkin JF, Marziali E, Munroe-Blum H. New York, Guilford, 1992, pp 3–23

Raine A: The Psychopathology of Crime: Criminal Behavior as a Clinical Disorder. San Diego, CA, Academic Press, 1993

Resnick MD, Bearman PS, Blum RW, et al: Protecting adolescents from harm: findings from the National Longitudinal Study of Adolescent Health. JAMA 278:823–832, 1997

Robins LN, Regier DA: Psychiatric Disorders in America: The Epidemiologic Catchment Area Study. New York, Free Press, 1991

Sher KJ, Trull TJ: Personality and disinhibitory psychopathology: alcoholism and antisocial personality disorder. J Abnorm Psychol 103:92–102, 1994

Skodol AE: Emergency management of potentially violent patients, in Emergency Psychiatry: Concepts, Methods, and Practices. Edited by Bassuk EL, Birk AW. New York, Plenum, 1984, pp 83–96

Skodol AE: Classification, assessment, and differential diagnosis of personality disorders. Journal of Practical Psychiatry and Behavioral Health 3:261–274, 1997

Skodol AE, Gallaher PE, Oldham JM: Aggression in borderlines seeking treatment. Paper presented at the annual meeting of the American Psychiatric Association, New York, NY, 1996

Stone MH: Treatment of severe personality disorders, in American Psychiatric Press Review of Psychiatry, Vol 11. Edited by Tasman A, Riba MB. Washington, DC, American Psychiatric Press, 1992, pp 98–115

Widiger TA, Trull TJ: Personality disorders and violence, in Violence and Mental Disorder: Developments in Risk Assessment. Edited by Monahan J, Steadman HJ. Chicago, IL, University of Chicago Press, 1994, pp 203–226

Index

Page numbers in **boldface** type refer to tables or figures.

Inpatients, studies relating violence to, 12–15

Jail inmates. *See* Prison inmates
Jealousy. *See* Pathological jealousy

Kaczynski, Theodore, 37
Karyotype, relation to crime and aggression, 104–105

Law, and psychopathology of crime, 129–131, 141–142
  legal response, 136–141
  legal views, 131–136
Lifetime Axis I mental disorders, in violent criminals, 65–66. *See also* Axis I mental disorders
  and criminal motivation, 68–74
  and index offenses, 67–68
  sexual deviation, 66–67

"Machiavellianism," 34
Manipulativeness, 34
Marshall, Rob, 47
McElroy, Ken, 36
Menendez brothers, 36
Mental disorders. *See* Axis I mental disorders; Axis II personality disorders; Law, and psychopathology of crime
Metabolic mediators, in crime and aggression studies, 112–115
Minns, Richard, 38–39
Murderers. *See also* Violent criminals
  personalities of, 29–30, 46–49
    antisocial, 31–32
    biographies as source material about, 30–31
    borderline, 40–42
    narcissistic, 35–36
    paranoid, 38–40
    psychopathic, 32–35
    schizoid, 37–38
    sadistic, 42–45
  studies relating mental disorders to, 5–6

Narcissistic personality disorder (NPD)
  and criminal motivation, 83–85

in murderers, 35–36
Neuropsychological dysfunction, as genesis of violent behavior, 17–18
Neurotransmitter mediators, in crime and aggression studies, 106–112
Nonculpability, implications of, 134–136
Norepinephrine, in crime and aggression studies, 110–111

Offenders. *See also* Violent criminals
  assessment of, 54–55
  violent, studies relating mental disorders to, 6–8
Outpatients, studies relating violence to, 15

Paranoid personality disorder
  and criminal motivation, 85
  in murderers, 38–40
Pathological jealousy, 38–39
Personality disorders. *See* Axis II personality disorders
Pierce, Darci, 42
Poddar, Prosenjit, 39, 40
Prison inmates, studies relating mental disorders to, 8–11. *See also* Violent criminals
Psychiatric patients, studies relating violence to
  case register study, 11–12
  delusional patient samples, 16–17
  inpatient samples, 12–15
  outpatient samples, 15
Psychopathic personality, in murderers, 32–35
Psychopathology. *See* Axis I mental disorders; Axis II personality disorders; Law, and psychopathology of crime

Remorse, lack of, 34, 43
Risk factors, biosocial, as genesis of violent behavior, 19–20
Ryan, Michael, 47